THE PSYCHOLOGY OF SPORT INJURY AND REHABILITATION

Athletes routinely use psychological interventions for performance enhancement but, perhaps surprisingly, not always to assist in recovery from injury. This book demonstrates the ways in which athletes and practitioners can transfer psychological skills to an injury and rehabilitation setting, to enhance recovery and the well-being of the athlete.

Drawing on the very latest research in sport and exercise psychology, this book explores key psychological concepts relating to injury, explaining typical psychological responses to injury and psychological aspects of rehabilitation. Using case studies in the chapters to highlight the day-to-day reality of working with injured athletes, it introduces a series of practical interventions, skills and techniques, underpinned by an evidence base, with a full explanation of how each might affect an athlete's recovery from injury.

The Psychology of Sport Injury and Rehabilitation emphasises the importance of a holistic, multi-disciplinary approach to sport injury and rehabilitation. No other book examines the psychological aspects of both sport injury and the rehabilitation process from such a holistic perspective, and therefore this is an essential resource for students, scholars and practitioners working in sport psychology, sport therapy, sport medicine or coaching.

Monna Arvinen-Barrow is a British Psychological Society chartered psychologist working as an Assistant Professor at the University of Wisconsin-Milwaukee, USA. Monna has a number of peer-reviewed publications on the psychology of sport injuries and has taught psychology of sport injuries in the United Kingdom, United States and Finland.

Natalie Walker is a British Psychological Society chartered/Health and Care Professions Council registered psychologist working as a Senior Lecturer at the University of Northampton, UK, and an Associate Lecturer at the Open University. Natalie has written a number of publications, as well as examining and supervising postgraduate/doctoral research in the area of the psychology of sport injuries.

THE PSYCHOLOGY OF SPORT INJURY AND REHABILITATION

Edited by Monna Arvinen-Barrow and Natalie Walker

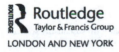

LONDON AND NEW YORK

First published 2013
by Routledge
2 Park Square, Milton Park, Abingdon, Oxon OX14 4RN

Simultaneously published in the USA and Canada
by Routledge
711 Third Avenue, New York, NY 10017

Routledge is an imprint of the Taylor and Francis Group, an informa business

British Library Cataloguing in Publication Data
A catalogue record for this book is available from the British Library

Library of Congress Cataloging in Publication Data
The psychology of sport injury and rehabilitation / edited by Monna Arvinen-
Barrow and Natalie Walker.
pages cm
1. Sports injuries–Psychological aspects. I. Arvinen-Barrow, Monna. II. Walker,
Natalie.
RD97.P79 2013
617.1'027–dc23
2012042544

ISBN: 978-0-415-69495-7 (hbk)
ISBN: 978-0-415-69589-3 (pbk)
ISBN: 978-0-203-55240-7 (ebk)

Typeset in Bembo
by FiSH Books Ltd, Enfield

Printed and bound in the United States of America by Edwards Brothers Malloy on sustainably sourced paper.

Äidin pienelle enkelille, Amielle (to Mommy's little angel, Amie) and in memory of my Dad. I wish you could have seen this in print.

Monna

To my family, I love you all so much Mum, Chris, Kieron, Ashleigh, Perry, Kaydee-Jayne, Maci-Ann, Keaton-Lee, Bailey and Ruby.

Natalie

CONTENTS

FIGURES AND TABLES

Figures

Tables

CONTRIBUTORS

Renee N. Appaneal is an Associate Professor in Kinesiology at the University of North Carolina at Greensboro, USA. In addition, Renee is a Certified Consultant with Association for Applied Sport Psychology, member of the US Olympic Committee's Sport Psychology Registry, and a Licensed Professional Counsellor (LPC) in North Carolina, USA. She consults with sport medicine professionals and other healthcare providers as well as provides sport and performance psychology services across a variety of settings and competitive athletic levels.

Monna Arvinen-Barrow is an Assistant Professor at University of Wisconsin-Milwaukee, USA. Monna recently moved to the USA from the UK, where she worked as a Senior Lecturer in Sport and Exercise Psychology at the University of Northampton and as an Associate Lecturer for the Open University. In addition to teaching sport and exercise psychology courses in the UK and US, Monna has also been teaching psychology of sport and exercise injury courses as a Visiting Scholar at the University of Jyväskylä, Finland. She is a British Psychological Society Chartered Psychologist, and an elected expert member of the Finnish Sport Psychology Association. She has a specialist interest and expertise in psychological rehabilitation from sport and exercise injuries and has completed her PhD entitled *Psychological Rehabilitation from Sports Injury: Issues in Training and Development of Chartered Physiotherapists* in 2009. In addition, she has published a number of peer-reviewed journal articles in the area of sport psychology, including several related to psychology of sport injury rehabilitation. Her sporting background comes from figure and synchronized skating where she has also been working as a professional coach for several years.

Britton W. Brewer is a Professor of Psychology at Springfield College in Springfield, Massachusetts, USA, where he teaches undergraduate and graduate psychology courses and conducts research on psychological aspects of sport injury.

Damien Clement is an Assistant Professor at West Virginia University's College of Physical Activity and Sport Sciences in Morgantown, USA, where he teaches undergraduate and graduate sport and exercise psychology courses and graduate athletic training courses. He is a Certified Athletic Trainer, National Certified Counselor, and Certified Consultant with Association for Applied Sport Psychology, as well as listed on the United States Olympic Committee Sport Psychology Registry.

Megan D. Granquist is an Assistant Professor of Movement and Sports Science at the University of La Verne in Southern California, USA. She teaches courses in sport psychology and kinesiology. She is a Certified Athletic Trainer and her research is focused on psychosocial factors related to sport injury and rehabilitation.

Stephanie Habif is a Lecturer at the Hasso Plattner Institute of Design at Stanford University in Palo Alto, California, USA. Stephanie conducts health behaviour change research with the Stanford Persuasive Technology and Calming Technology Labs, provides performance psychology services to injured and obese people, and consults with health technology start-ups and healthcare corporations.

J. Jordan Hamson-Utley is an Assistant Professor and director of athletic training education programme at Weber State University, Ogden, Utah, USA, where she continues her research on examining the effects of psychological strategies on physiological biomarkers associated with symptom resolution and return to play in injured athletes. Jordan is also a certified athletic trainer who gained her PhD in Experimental Psychology, where she implemented various cognitive interventions with athletes rehabilitating from sport injury. She has worked with athletes from all levels, including the US men's and women's soccer teams and Olympic athletes at the Olympic Training Center in Colorado Springs and the Pan Am Games in Santo Domingo (2003).

Elaine A. Hargreaves is a Senior Lecturer in Exercise and Sport Psychology at the University of Otago, New Zealand. Her research is focused on understanding the motivational forces behind the decision to adopt and maintain a physically active lifestyle.

Caroline Heaney is a Senior Lecturer in Sport and Exercise Science at the Open University, UK. She is a British Association of Sport and Exercise Sciences accredited and Health and Care Professions Council registered Sport Psychologist. Caroline has provided sport psychology support to a wide range of performers.

Brian Hemmings is a Consultant Sport Psychologist and a Visiting Researcher at the School of Human Sciences, St. Mary's University College, Twickenham, UK. Brian is a British Psychological Society Chartered Psychologist, and a Health and

Care Professions Council Registered Sport and Exercise Psychologist working full-time in private practice. Brian has worked extensively with a range of Olympic, professional and amateur sports for twenty years and is currently involved with élite performers in international golf, cricket and motorsport.

Joanne Hudson is Head of the Department of Sport and Exercise Science and a Senior Lecturer in Sport and Exercise Psychology at Aberystwyth University, UK. She is British Psychological Society Chartered Psychologist and Associate Fellow, as well as British Association of Sport and Exercise Sciences accredited and Health and Care Professions Council Registered. She has co-authored and co-edited four texts on sport and exercise science and psychology and has published in a number of national and international peer-reviewed journals.

Jonathan Katz is a Consultant Psychologist working full time in private practice. Jonathan is a British Psychological Society Chartered Psychologist and Associate Fellow, as well as Health and Care Professions Council Registered. Jonathan has provided psychological coaching support to a range of individuals (athletes, coaches, managers and performance directors), competing at national and international levels including World Cup Events, European and World Championships and Commonwealth, Olympic and Paralympic Games across a wide range of individual, team, amateur and professional sports. He was also the Great Britain Head Quarters Psychologist for ParalympicsGB at both the Athens 2004 and Beijing 2008 Summer Paralympic Games and the lead psychologist for the Turin 2006 Winter Paralympic Games. He has also been the team psychologist to the British Disabled Ski Team at the Vancouver 2010 Winter Paralympic Games and squad psychologist for Disability Target Shooting GB at the London 2012 Summer Paralympic Games.

Cindra S. Kamphoff is an Associate Professor in Sport and Exercise Psychology at Minnesota State University, Mankato, USA. Cindra is a Certified Consultant with the Association for Applied Sport Psychology and serves on the AASP Executive Committee. She works with all athletes and performers, and specialises in the psychology of running. She enjoys running marathons in her spare time.

Stephen Pack is a Senior Lecturer in Sport and Exercise Psychology at the University of Hertfordshire, UK. Stephen is a British Psychological Society Chartered Psychologist, is Health and Care Professions Council registered, as well as being accredited by the British Association of Sport and Exercise Sciences. He has worked with athletes and performers in a variety of contexts including archery, cycling, golf, and polar exploration.

Jeffrey Thomae is an instructor in the Department of Human Performance at Minnesota State University, Mankato, USA, teaching courses in both sport psychology and sport sociology. In addition, Jeffrey is a Performance Consultant for the Center for Sport and Performance Psychology at MSU, Mankato, drawing on experience in coaching, counseling, and mental skills training to assist athletes, coaches, exercisers, and performing artists alike.

Natalie Walker is a Senior Lecturer in Sport and Exercise Psychology at the University of Northampton and an Associate Lecturer for the Open University, UK. Natalie is a British Psychological Society Chartered and Health and Care Professions Council Registered Sport and Exercise Psychologist. Natalie also works as an applied sport psychology consultant to various sporting individuals and teams. She has a specialist interest and expertise in psychological rehabilitation from sport injuries and has completed her PhD entitled *The Meaning of Sports Injury and Re-injury Anxiety Assessment and Intervention* in 2006. In addition, she has a number of peer-reviewed journal and book chapter publications in this area, and has also examined postgraduate theses related to psychology of injuries and is currently supervising PhDs in this field. Her sporting background comes from association football and martial arts.

Julie A. Waumsley is a Senior Lecturer and Course Leader for the undergraduate and postgraduate degree programmes in counselling at The University of Northampton, UK. Julie's expertise in counselling and performance issues is relevant in the sport domain, where she is a British Psychological Society Chartered and Health and Care Professions Council registered Sport and Exercise Psychologist. Her background is in sport and leisure, having spent ten years as an Army Physical Training Instructor and ten years in leisure management before embarking on her academic career.

FOREWORD

A book on the psychology of sport injuries is not groundbreaking. I start with this not as a criticism but as an acknowledgement of how this area of study has advanced in recent years. In 1993, two edited texts which could be described as groundbreaking were published in this area, namely *Psychological Bases of Sport Injuries* (edited by David Pargman and published by Fitness Information Technology) and *Psychology of Sport Injury* (edited by John Heil and published by Human Kinetics). These books were the first to focus on sport injuries purely from a psychological perspective to assist practitioners in working with athletes. They were highly successful in reviewing material at the time. Considering the respective content lists of the two 1993 texts alongside the current edition by Monna Arvinen-Barrow and Natalie Walker shows how much has advanced over the past 20 years. Indeed, the preface in Pargman's 1993 text noted how its goal was to provide 'caveats and clues' to practitioners (and those preparing for such careers) in the field. The current edition is able to draw on a far more diverse and established literature and thus to provide clearer evidence-based recommendations with regard to sport injury and rehabilitation.

A consequence of having a greater breath of coverage is the challenge of not neglecting anything in one volume. The Editors have chosen their chapter authors well, as they have collectively delivered on this challenge. The book impressively considers relevant psychological theories (behavioural, cognitive, developmental, personality, humanist, social psychology and learning theories), major psychological concepts (cognition, attention, emotion, motivation, personality, behaviour, anxiety, interpersonal relationships) and takes into account relevant groups who influence and are influenced by sport injuries (athletes, coaches, psychologists, parents, friends, organisations, doctors, physiotherapist, lifestyle advisors, team mates and others).

The accessibility of *The Psychology of Sport Injury and Rehabilitation* for a range of professionals is one of its greatest strengths. Case studies and testimonies allow the reader to appreciate and understand the sport experience from the athlete's perspective. Although it was not the objective of the Editors to bring conclusions to the debates associated with how injuries are defined, the book makes a strong case for psychology to be explicitly referred to in such definitions. Without doubt, the book will help further promote interest in the area and stimulate work over the next 20 years and beyond.

David Lavallee
University of Stirling

PREFACE

Monna Arvinen-Barrow and Natalie Walker

> *I just expect to be able to play...back at the level that I was before I think... just... just to go back to what I did before, I think you just want to be back and able to do what you did before the injury.*
>
> *(An injured association football player)*

The sport injury experience from an athlete's perspective is as diverse as the number of athletes sustaining injuries and types of injuries encountered. Each injury experience is unique, and is influenced by a range of personal and situational biopsychosocial factors that interact not only during but also before and after the injury occurrence. Nevertheless, the above quote in its simplicity may summarise the key hopes and dreams of those injured – to be able to return back to pre-injury levels of function.

As varied as the injury experiences themselves is the terminology surrounding the sport injury literature, research and applied work. For example, sport injuries still lack a unified definition but, given that there are a number of ways in which sport injuries can be classified, such may not be surprising. It is not our aim to bring conclusions to such debates but rather to adopt one view from which this book has been written. As such, for the purposes of this book, sport (and physical activity) injuries will be defined as 'trauma to the body or its parts that result in at least temporary, but sometimes permanent physical disability and inhibition of motor function' (Berger, Pargman and Weinberg, 2007: 186).

Based on the definition above, we see sport injuries as being physical in nature, which, depending on severity, may require assistance from medical professionals to ensure appropriate healing and recovery. To expand the applicability of the content presented in this book across different cultures, in this book, we have adopted the term *sport medicine professionals* as an overarching title for all those working with injured athletes. This can include (but is not limited to) all those required to assist the injured athlete to return to their pre-injury level physically and psychologically: the physiotherapist, athletic trainer, sport therapist, massage therapist, orthopaedic surgeon, other medical doctors, sport (and exercise) psychologist, counselling and clinical psychologist, psychiatrist, counsellor and other allied health professionals.

Throughout the book, we address the notion that sport injuries, despite being physical in nature, also have psychological facets. It is also believed that psychological skills (that is, mental abilities of athletes) can assist athletes in the rehabilitation process. These skills can be facilitated and enhanced through the use of psychological techniques (that is, methods an athlete can use to rehearse or improve psychological skills). For the purposes of this book, when referring to these psychological techniques (for example, goal setting, imagery, relaxation techniques, self-talk and social support) collectively, the term *psychological interventions* will be used. The book is also underpinned by the notion that psychological interventions are most successful if used as part of a wider rehabilitation programme incorporating a number of aspects deemed important for successful recovery. When discussing the term *rehabilitation* in this book, we consider it to include the treatment provided during all of the different phases of rehabilitation, from the injury onset through the rehabilitation process and up to and including the return to training and competition (including minimising the risk of re-injury). It is also believed that the use of psychological interventions should only be facilitated by professionals who are appropriately trained and skilled to do so.

To assist those interested in learning how to incorporate psychology into the sport injury process, this book demonstrates ways in which this might be achieved. We provide some suggestions as to how sport medicine professionals may amalgamate physical and psychological rehabilitation for it to become an accepted part of a holistic sport injury rehabilitation process, rather than an addition to it. More specifically, the book provides a contemporary overview of the subject area from experts within the field from across the world. The objective of this book is to offer scholars and practitioners alike a text that they will not only find invaluable in terms of knowledge gained but unique and contemporary in terms of practice.

To this end, this book is divided into three parts. Part 1, 'Introduction to the psychology of sport injuries: theoretical frameworks', introduces the key terminology, theories and models used in the book, and highlights the importance of addressing psychological issues during rehabilitation to ensure a full and holistic recovery. More specifically, Chapter 1 provides the reader with a rationale for the book by introducing the concept of psychology of sport injuries, and by providing awareness of the importance of psychology in the sport injury process. Chapter 2 provides an overview of psychological and social factors that can contribute to the onset of injury. It outlines Andersen and Williams' (1988) pre-injury model and provides a summary of a contemporary systematic review of the literature explaining psychological factors affecting the incidence of sport injury. Moreover, the chapter highlights the importance of understanding pre-injury factors in relation to sport injury rehabilitation and the ways in which these factors can help to facilitate or, in some cases, hinder any subsequent rehabilitation. Chapter 3 then provides a critical overview of the models of response to injury to date. The major focus of the chapter is on the integrated model of response to sports injury and rehabilitation (Wiese-Bjornstal, Smith, Shaffer and Morrey, 1998) with a discussion of its application to real-life injury rehabilitation on a more practical level. This model serves as a foundation for subsequent chapters as, within the model, the idea of interactions between injured athletes' cognitive appraisals, emotional responses and behavioural responses can be used as a framework when designing rehabilitation programmes and choosing appropriate psychological interventions to meet the injured athletes' needs. Chapter 4 concludes Part 1 by outlining adherence to sport injury rehabilitation as a prime area of interest in the psychology of sport injury. As adherence issues are seen as one of the main influences on athletes not recovering successfully, this chapter highlights the importance of addressing adherence during rehabilitation, and thus provides a rationale for Part 2 of the book, 'Psychological interventions in sport injury rehabilitation'.

Part 2 has its focus on the five most popular psychological interventions (goal setting, imagery, relaxation techniques, self-talk and social support). Presented in five distinct chapters, each of the interventions is introduced by discussing the key concepts and demonstrating their usefulness and applicability to sport injury rehabilitation. Each chapter discusses the theoretical underpinnings of the intervention and their use for promoting holistic recovery.

Part 3, 'Delivering psychological interventions in sport injury rehabilitation' introduces the reader to some of the practicalities of integrating psychological and physical rehabilitation. More specifically, Chapter 10 demonstrates the relationship between different phases of physical rehabilitation and how to use rehabilitation profiling as a foundation for designing, planning and implementing appropriate psychological interventions alongside physical rehabilitation. Following on, Chapter 11 highlights the importance of multidisciplinary teams and the integration of sport medicine professionals and significant others as part of psychological rehabilitation from sport injuries. Chapter 12 then discusses the ways in which basic counselling skills could also be beneficial in assisting sport injury rehabilitation. Chapter 13 applies the existing knowledge of psychology of sport injuries in the context of physical activity related injuries, taking into account the differences in personal and situational factors between sport and physical activity participants. Moreover, the possible impact of physical activity related injuries on an individual's future participation will be discussed (such as barriers to physical activity). Finally, Chapter 14 provides conclusions on the psychological processes of sport injury rehabilitation. It draws on the chapters presented in the three distinct parts of the book and summarises the existing knowledge, as well as provides some broad over-arching recommendations for applied work, and future research in the field.

Chapters 2–13 are also enhanced with individual case studies specifically focusing on the issues presented in the corresponding chapter. These case studies are accompanied by questions that are aimed to assist the reader to explore their understanding of the theory and application of the topic discussed. The link between theory and practice will be further enhanced through the use of real-life quotes from sport medicine professionals and injured athletes alike. Moreover, each of the chapters will also highlight some of the key points to be drawn from the chapter by framing them within the text. By doing so, this book aims to provide the reader with a comprehensive view of the process of psychological rehabilitation from sport injuries, by adopting a holistic perspective incorporating theory, research, and applied knowledge.

References

Andersen, M. B. and Williams, J. M. (1988) A model of stress and athletic injury: prediction and prevention. *Journal of Sport and Exercise Psychology*, 10, 294–306.

Berger, B. G., Pargman, D. and Weinberg, R. S. (2007) *Foundations of exercise psychology*, 2nd edn. Morgantown, WV: Fitness Information Technology.

Wiese-Bjornstal, D. M., Smith, A. M., Shaffer, S. M. and Morrey, M. A. (1998) An integrated model of response to sport injury: Psychological and sociological dynamics. *Journal of Applied Sport Psychology*, 10, 46–69.

ACKNOWLEDGEMENTS

It is with great appreciation that we thank several people for playing central roles in the completion of this book. First, our sincere gratitude goes to the authors of each chapter, who produced thoughtful and significant contributions in a timely manner throughout the process. Without your wealth of expertise in this field, this book would not have been possible, so many thanks for going the extra mile and making the editorial process 'injury' free.

We would also like to say a very special thank you to Dr Julie Waumsley. Both of us are greatly indebted to your initial spark for the idea of this book and for maintaining momentum in the initial stages. Moreover, we thank you for your valuable time in making important early contributions to the administrative and structural aspects of the book in addition to co-authoring two chapters.

We are also indebted to Stephen Worrall for giving up his time to review each chapter in detail and provide comprehensive feedback – and for making sure our apostrophes are now in right places!

Finally, our gratitude is extended to Routledge for commissioning the book. In particular, we would like to thank Joshua Wells and Simon Whitmore for being invaluable in guiding us throughout the publication process.

Monna and Natalie

I would like to say *KIITOS* to all of my academic friends and colleagues who have had an impact on my career. Natalie, thank you for six great years working together, it has been fun. A special acknowledgement goes to my dear friend/mentor/colleague Dr Brian Hemmings. Thank you for your continued support and guidance, and for always believing in me. A huge thank you goes to my family, who never fail to support me in my crazy endeavours like moving across the world or editing a book. In particular, *ISO KIITOS* to my little angel Amie. The power of your smile always keeps me going.

Monna

I would like to thank those in academia who I have had the pleasure of working with. Particular thanks to Nichola Kentzer, who has been my sounding board for the latter part of this book. Of course, a huge thank you goes to my co-editor, Monna. We have shared an office for six years and have ended our office sharing by completing this book. What a way to end! I wish you the very best overseas. Thanks also to Dr Jo Hudson: you have played a significant role in shaping my academic career and for that I will always be grateful. Finally, I must thank my amazing family. Mum, you have always believed in me and I hope I continue to make you proud, I love you so much. Chris, Kieron, Ashleigh, Perry, Kaydee-Jayne, Maci-Ann and Keaton-Lee, you are my world and thanks for always being there and believing in me.

Natalie

INTRODUCTION TO THE
PSYCHOLOGY OF SPORT INJURIES

PART 1

Introduction to the psychology of sport injuries: theoretical frameworks

1

INTRODUCTION TO THE PSYCHOLOGY OF SPORT INJURIES

Monna Arvinen-Barrow and Natalie Walker

In society today, sport can form an important part of the ways in which an individual identifies themselves, how they interact with one another and reflect on their position amongst those around them. According to the Council of Europe (2001), the term sport refers to 'all forms of physical activity which, through casual or organised participation, aim at expressing or improving physical fitness and mental well-being, forming social relationships or obtaining results in competition at all levels'. At its best, sport can provide opportunities for physical, psychological and economic growth, and be a vehicle for providing exciting, challenging, rewarding and memorable experiences for all those involved. Despite such positive benefits, unfortunately some experiences gained through sport are in fact the opposite (Brown, 2005). Involvement in sport frequently places the participants under immense physical and psychological pressure and stress, which in turn amplifies the likelihood of negative outcomes, such as injuries. Although injuries are an experience that athletes are trying to avoid (Pargman, 1999), virtually all athletes will experience an injury that can temporarily (or permanently) impede any subsequent sport participation (Taylor and Taylor, 1997). In fact, Brown (2005) argues that 'serious athletes come in two varieties: those who have been injured, and those who have not been injured yet'.

Such a claim is supported in the literature. For example, in Australia, it has been estimated that 20 per cent of all child/adolescent and 18 per cent of adult hospital accident and emergency room consultations were sport injury related (Finch, Valuri and Ozanne-Smith, 1998). In 2002, approximately 20.3 million Americans suffered a sport injury, of which half required medical attention (Conn, Annest and Gilchrist, 2003). In the UK, it has been estimated that nearly 30 million sport-related injuries occur every year (Nicholl, Coleman and Williams, 1995), accounting for nearly 33 per cent of all injuries nationwide (Uitenbroek, 1996). More recently, in Finland, it was found that amongst adolescent male and female athletes involved in association football, ice hockey, basketball, cross-country skiing, figure skating, gymnastics and athletics, 50.4 per cent of all that responded reported having suffered sport-related injuries in the past 12 months (Konttinen, Mononen, Pihlaja, Sipari, Arvinen-Barrow and Selänne, 2011).

With the aid of advanced medical knowledge and technology, most injured athletes have the potential for full recovery to their pre-injury (or in some cases higher) level of fitness and performance. However, numerous athletes fail to recover back to their pre-injury level of play (Taylor and Taylor, 1997) and often this failure is attributable to psychological factors. It has been highlighted that psychological factors can influence injury onset and can also determine the extent to which an athlete is able to cope successfully with injury and its subsequent rehabilitation (see, for example, Arvinen-Barrow, Hemmings, Weigand, Becker and Booth, 2007; Clement, Granquist and Arvinen-Barrow, 2013; Heaney, 2006; Hemmings and Povey, 2002; Larson, Starkey and Zaichkowsky, 1996). Furthermore, research has also found links between sport injuries and reduced levels of self-esteem, loss of personal identity, anxiety (for example, pre-injury anxiety; Walker, 2006), depression and, on occasions, feelings of isolation (Leddy, Lambert and Ogles, 1994; Petitpas and Danish, 1995).

Drawing from existing sport injury literature, it is apparent that both physical and psychological factors can have a significant impact on sport injury susceptibility, injury occurrence, cognitive appraisals of injury, emotional and behavioural responses to the injury, the overall injury recovery outcomes and the return to sport (see, for example, Ievleva and Orlick, 1991; McDonald and Hardy, 1990; Wiese-Bjornstal, Smith, Shaffer and Morrey, 1998). It has also been suggested that the use of psychological interventions can be beneficial in the context of sport injuries as they have the potential to: (a) reduce athletes injury susceptibility (Williams and Andersen, 1998), (b) facilitate injury recovery (Ievleva and Orlick, 1991), (c) provide a sense of control over the rehabilitation process subsequently enhancing motivation and rehabilitation adherence (Flint, 1998), and (d) increase communication between the athlete and the medical professional working with the athlete (Ray and Wiese-Bjornstal, 1999). These can facilitate injured athletes' greater understanding of the injury, the injury process and possible recovery outcomes (Heaney, 2006; Hemmings and Povey, 2002). A greater understanding of the injury can also affect treatment compliance, which is also believed to have an effect on athletes' coping skills and injury recovery (see, for example, Arvinen-Barrow et al., 2007; Hemmings and Povey, 2002). Moreover, athletes who engage in psychological interventions which enable them to perceive themselves as active agents in their recovery are more likely to have better physical recovery outcomes (Durso-Cupal, 1996).

The most popular and prominent psychological interventions used in sport today are goal setting, imagery, relaxation training and positive self-talk (Brown, 2005; Vealey, 1988). Encouraging and employing the use of social support has also been identified as important and beneficial for injured athletes (Brown, 2005; Heil, 1993). However, despite the widely accepted view that all of the above psychological interventions are extremely useful in assisting athletes to achieve performance gains, they are often underused in sport injury prevention and rehabilitation by both the injured athlete and the medical professionals alike (see, for example, Arvinen-Barrow, Penny, Hemmings and Corr, 2010).

Such underuse could be attributable to number of reasons. Firstly, it has been proposed that both athletes and sport medicine professionals working with injured athletes may be unable to transfer existing skills from performance enhancement settings to the injury rehabilitation context. Secondly, those working with injured athletes may possess limited knowledge on how to use psychological interventions during injury rehabilitation, as it appears that only a few professionals have been extensively trained to use such skills during sport injury rehabilitation. For example, in the UK, physiotherapy educators profess to deliver their psychology content through an integrated approach, with a view that this approach would lead to a more applied understanding of the topic. However, there is often a disparity between knowledge of the subject and the ability to apply this knowledge to benefit individuals (Heaney, Green, Rostron and Walker, 2012). Thirdly, it may be that psychological interventions are underused simply because of lack of adequate understanding of how psychological interventions can be integrated seamlessly into physical rehabilitation. As such, the principle aim of this book is to demonstrate ways in which psychology plays a role in the sport injury process and how psychological interventions can be used in sport injury rehabilitation. After all, by attending to the psychological needs of the athlete, the practitioners working with injured athletes are treating the whole person, and not just the injury, and thus offering a more holistic approach to recovery.

References

Arvinen-Barrow, M., Hemmings, B., Weigand, D. A., Becker, C. A. and Booth, L. (2007) Views of chartered physiotherapists on the psychological content of their practice: A national follow-up survey in the United Kingdom. *Journal of Sport Rehabilitation*, 16, 111–121.

Arvinen-Barrow, M., Penny, G., Hemmings, B. and Corr, S. (2010) UK Chartered Physiotherapists' personal experiences in using psychological interventions with injured athletes: an interpretative phenomenological analysis. *Psychology of Sport and Exercise*, 11, 58–66.

Brown, C. (2005) Injuries: The psychology of recovery and rehab. In S. Murphy (ed.), *The sport psych handbook*. Champaign, IL: Human Kinetics, pp. 215–35.

Clement, D., Granquist, M. and Arvinen-Barrow, M. (2013) Psychosocial aspects of athletic injuries as perceived by athletic trainers. *Journal of Athletic Training*.

Conn, J. M., Annest, J. L. and Gilchrist, J. (2003) Sports and recreation related injury episodes in the US population, 1997–99. *Injury Prevention*, 9(2), 117–23.

Council of Europe. (2001) *The European Sports Charter (revised)*. Brussels: Council of Europe. Retrieved from http://www.sportdevelopment.info/index.php/subjects/59-international-documents/87-council-of-europe-2001-the-european-sports-charterrevised-brussels-council-of-europe-

Durso-Cupal, D. (1996) The efficacy of guided imagery for recovery from anterior cruciate ligament (ACL) replacement. *Journal of Applied Sport Psychology*, 8(suppl), S56.

Finch, C., Valuri, G. and Ozanne-Smith, J. (1998) Sport and active recreation injuries in Australia: evidence from emergency department presentations. *British Journal of Sports Medicine*, 32(3), 220–5.

Flint, F. A. (1998) Specialized psychological interventions In F. A. Flint (ed.), *Psychology of Sport Injury*. Leeds: Human Kinetics, pp. 29–50.

Heaney, C. (2006) Physiotherapists' perceptions of sport psychology intervention in professional soccer. *International Journal of Sport and Exercise Psychology*, 4(1), 67–80.

Heaney, C., Green, A. J. K., Rostron, C. L. and Walker, N. (2012) A qualitative and quantitative investigation of the psychology content of UK physiotherapy education programs. *Journal of Physical Therapy Education*.

Heil, J. (1993) *Psychology of Sport Injury*. Champaign, IL: Human Kinetics.

Hemmings, B. and Povey, L. (2002) Views of chartered physiotherapists on the psychological content of their practice: A preliminary study in the United Kingdom. *British Journal of Sports Medicine*, 36, 61–4.

Ievleva, L. and Orlick, T. (1991) Mental links to enhanced healing: An exploratory study. *The Sport Psychologist*, 5, 25–40.

Konttinen, N., Mononen, K., Pihlaja, T., Sipari, T., Arvinen-Barrow, M. and Selänne, H. (2011) Urheiluvammojen esiintyminen ja niiden hoito nuorisourheilussa – Kohderyhmänä 1995 syntyneet urheilijat. [Sport injury occurence and treatment in youth sports – athletes born in 1995 as a target population]. *KIHUn julkaisusarja nro 25 (PDF-julkaisu)*, 1–16. Retrieved from http://www.kihu.jyu.fi/tuotokset/haku/index.php?hae=Tee+haku#TOC2011.

Larson, G. A., Starkey, C. and Zaichkowsky, L. D. (1996) Psychological aspects of athletic injuries as perceived by athletic trainers. *The Sport Psychologist*, 10, 37–47.

Leddy, M. H., Lambert, M. J. and Ogles, B. M. (1994) Psychological consequences of athletic injury among high level competitors. *Research Quarterly for Exercise and Sport*, 65, 347–54.

McDonald, S. A. and Hardy, C. J. (1990) Affective response patterns of the injured athlete: An exploratory analysis. *The Sport Psychologist*, 4, 261–74.

Nicholl, J. P., Coleman, P. and Williams, B. T. (1995) The epidemiology of sports and exercise related injury in the United Kingdom. *British Journal of Sports Medicine*, 29, 232–38.

Pargman, D. (ed.) (1999) *Psychological Bases of Sport Injuries*, 2nd edn. Morgantown, WV: Fitness Information Technology Inc.

Petitpas, A. and Danish, S. J. (1995) Caring for injured athletes. In S. Murphy (ed.), *Sport Psychology Interventions*. Champaign, IL: Human Kinetics, pp. 255–81.

Ray, R. and Wiese-Bjornstal, D. M. (eds). (1999) *Counseling in Sports Medicine*. Champaign, IL: Human Kinetics.

Taylor, J. and Taylor, S. (1997) *Psychological Approaches to Sports Injury Rehabilitation*. Gaithersburg, MD: Aspen.

Uitenbroek, D. G. (1996) Sports, exercise, and other causes of injuries: Results of a population survey. *Research Quarterly for Exercise and Sport*, 67, 380–5.

Vealey, R. S. (1988) Future directions in psychological skills training. *The Sport Psychologist*, 2(4), 318–336.

Walker, N. (2006) *The Meaning of Sports Injury and Re-injury Anxiety Assessment and Intervention*. (Unpublished PhD dissertation), University of Wales, Aberystwyth.

Wiese-Bjornstal, D. M., Smith, A. M., Shaffer, S. M. and Morrey, M. A. (1998) An integrated model of response to sport injury: Psychological and sociological dynamics. *Journal of Applied Sport Psychology*, 10, 46–69.

Williams, J. M. and Andersen, M. B. (1998) Psychosocial antecedents of sport injury: Review and critique of the stress and injury model. *Journal of Sport and Exercise Psychology*, 10, 5–25.

2

PSYCHOLOGICAL ANTECEDENTS TO SPORT INJURY

Renee N. Appaneal and Stephanie Habif

Introduction

Sport-related injuries are a significant public health concern for physically active individuals (Centers for Disease Control and Prevention, 2002; Conn, Annest and Gilchrist, 2003; Marshall and Guskiewicz, 2003). As a result, it is not surprising that sport injury surveillance and prevention efforts have included national and organisational monitoring systems, safer equipment and playing environments and policies. Yet, among those widespread changes, psychological factors are rarely considered within comprehensive sport injury prevention recommendations (Engebretsen and Bahr, 2009). Derived from work conducted in the stress-illness domain, initial evidence for the stress–injury relationship came from two key studies in the 1970s (Bramwell, Masuda, Wagner and Holmes, 1975; Holmes, 1970). Both studies conducted psychological screenings with football players and found that the greater the stress, the greater the likelihood of injury. Studies were later replicated with American collegiate football players and their results yielded significant associations between life stress and sport injury (Coddington and Troxell, 1980; Cryan and Alles, 1983; Passer and Seese, 1983). However, findings from studies with other sports such as volleyball failed to demonstrate a relationship between life stress and injury (Williams, Tonymon and Wadsworth, 1986). In reviewing this body of research, Andersen and Williams (1988) noted the inconsistency and atheoretical nature of this work and offered a potentially unifying framework for psychological prediction and prevention of sport injury.

To ensure continued participation in sport and physical activity while minimising the risk of sport-related injury, it is important to understand psychological factors which may predispose an individual to injury. Therefore, the purpose of this chapter is to outline the psychological factors that are seen to be influencing the onset of sport injury. The chapter is based on the authors' own systematic review of 70 published and unpublished studies which examined the relationship between psychosocial factors and sport injury outcomes among competitive athletes between 1965 and 2009 (Appaneal, Habif, Washington and Granquist, 2009). More specifically, this chapter (a) introduces the stress and injury model (Andersen and Williams, 1988; Williams and Andersen, 1998); (b) reviews the different antecedents associated with athlete's stress response; (c) highlights the role of stress–response mechanisms in increasing sport injury occurrence; (d) summarises the evidence supporting the use of psychological interventions to prevent sport injuries; and (e) throughout the different sections of the chapter, suggests practical strategies for those wishing to translate this knowledge into professional practice (for example, for sport/performance psychology and sport medicine professionals).

The stress and injury model

The model of stress and injury (Andersen and Williams, 1988) was developed to organise research and direct future interest by explaining the psychology underlying the occurrence of sport injuries. According to the model, the likelihood of injury will be influenced by an athlete's perception of stress in a given situation. The model presumes that an athlete's personality, stress history, and coping resources all influence the athlete's cognitive appraisal of stress, which may either intensify or mitigate their response to stress within the athletic environment and subsequently enhance their risk of sustaining an injury. The cognitive appraisal process plays a key role in stress reactivity and involves a balance (or imbalance) between two individually based perceptions, the primary and secondary appraisals (Lazarus and Folkman, 1984). Both of these perceptions are largely subconscious and dynamic, where the primary appraisal reflects the perception of a stressor (or event) as threatening and/or harmful and having important consequences. The secondary appraisal involves the degree to which s/he perceives having adequate coping resources to manage the demands of that stressor. The basic premise of this model, then, is that athletes who have a personality that amplifies stress, history of many stressors and few available or effective coping resources to buffer stress, are more likely to have cognitive appraisals of athletic situations that heighten their stress responses and increase their risk of sustaining an injury. For example, athletes who appraise stressors as threatening/harmful and perceive a lack of adequate coping resources will likely experience heightened stress reactivity, which in turn influences physiological/attentional functioning. Stress-related impairments may include, but are not limited to, increased muscle tension, peripheral narrowing, and/or increased distractibility. The first may result in poor coordination of movement and the latter two may result in poor cue recognition, delayed decision making, increased reaction time or other sensorimotor disruptions. For athletes, according to this model, consequences of heightened stress reactivity experienced within a sporting environment, increases their risk of injury.

In addition to identifying factors guiding sport injury prediction, the stress and injury model (Andersen and Williams, 1988) also included potential psychological interventions to assist athletes in adapting to stress, which might serve to prevent sport injury from occurring. The intervention strategies reflect a cognitive behavioural approach to stress management (Meichenbaum, 1977), where skills training and support is provided to develop effective cognitive appraisals (for example, thought stopping, cognitive restructuring) and enhance personal control over various physiological/attentional effects of stress (such as relaxation, mental rehearsal, attention control training).

After Andersen and Williams (1988) proposed their framework, not surprisingly, research proliferated examining various aspects of the stress–injury model. A decade later, Williams and Andersen (1998) provided an updated review of the literature and proposed several revisions to their original model. These changes included the addition of several bidirectional arrows (that is, between personality and stress history, between stress history and coping resources, and between coping resources and personality). The changes also included limiting the model to explain the process of prediction and prevention of acute injuries and not chronic or overuse injuries, which were seen as likely to involve different stress–response processes (Williams and Andersen, 1998). Figure 2.1 displays an amalgamation of the original (Andersen and Williams, 1988) and the revised (Williams and Andersen, 1998) stress and injury models.

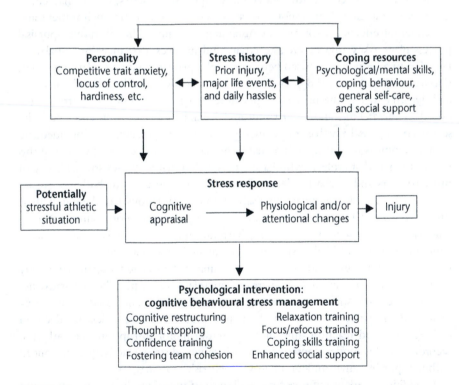

FIGURE 2.1 An amalgamated version of the stress and injury model

Source: adapted from Andersen and Williams' (1988) original model and Williams and Andersen's (1998) revised model

Drawing from the existing literature, it can be argued that, although the stress and injury model was introduced over 20 years ago, it still remains the single most dominant framework guiding today's research in psychology of sport injury prediction and prevention. The following sections discuss each of the components of the model in more detail by (a) reviewing the research conducted to date and (b) providing applied suggestions on the implications of such findings to those working with athletes.

In stressful athletic situations, individuals with certain personality characteristics (such as trait anxiety), high levels of stress and few coping resources (for example, lack of social support) appraise the situation as potentially threatening and perceive an inability to manage demands. As a result, those athletes will likely exhibit heightened stress reactivity, reflected by poor physiological (for example, increased muscle tension) and/or attentional functioning (for example, peripheral narrowing, increased distractibility), which, in turn, places them at greater risk of incurring athletic injury.

The stress response

According to the stress and injury model, stress responses may involve disruptions in athletes' cognitive/attentional and physiological functioning. In our review of the literature, we found only seven studies that were inclusive of both the stress responses and antecedents. Of those that did, stress responses were typically measured through athletes' perceptions of stress-related vulnerability, reaction time and attentional/visual indices (Andersen and Williams, 1999; Bergandi and Witting, 1988; Dahlhauser and Thomas, 1979; Dvorak et al., 2000; Kleinert, 2007; Rogers and Landers, 2005; Thompson and Morris, 1994). The results from these studies indicate that some of the factors contributing to poor stress response which may have facilitated a higher risk of sport injury include: low perceptions of health (may reflect either low resistance to stress or low confidence; Kleinert, 2007); slower reaction times (Dvorak et al., 2000) and peripheral narrowing (Andersen and Williams, 1999; Rogers and Landers, 2005). More specifically, peripheral narrowing was found to mediate the relationship between injury outcomes and high stress in college athletes (Andersen and Williams, 1999) and negative life stress in high-school athletes (Rogers and Landers, 2005). Further support (Bergandi and Witting, 1988; Dahlhauser and Thomas, 1979; Thompson and Morris, 1994) for the association between injury and visual/attentional aspects has also been documented among both high-school and college athletes and therefore supports the multidimensional nature of athletes' stress responses as outlined in the revised stress and injury model.

Impact of stress response research on injury occurrence: implications for sport medicine professionals

When working with athletes, sport medicine professionals should consider educating athletes about the importance of stress management and a healthy lifestyle (such as training, recovery, nutrition and sleep) for minimising the risk of sport injury. Athletes and coaches should be informed that, by balancing stress and recovery and consistently eating and sleeping well, they can minimise sensorimotor impairments and maintain energy and alertness, which in turn may promote health, support training adaptation, and enhance sport performance.

Antecedents of sport injury

As identified above, stress reactivity is the central link between stress and injury incidence. In the attempt to prevent injuries occurring, the principal aim of any psychological injury prevention efforts should be to determine what factors influence athletes' stress responses (Williams and Andersen, 1998, 2007). While there are three main factors identified in the model (personality, stress history and coping resources), each encompasses a variety of specific variables. Further, these variables are seen as antecedents influencing sport injury onset, in that that they precede stressful encounters in sport. They also reflect both risk factors and resources, in that they may buffer and/or or heighten athletes' stress reactivity and subsequent sport injury risk. To date, a breadth of research has examined psychological antecedents to sport injury. In our review, 65 of the 70 studies explored psychological factors associated with sport injury risk and 86 per cent of those reported significant findings between one or more risk factors and sport injury outcomes. The following sections provide a brief review of the literature, examining each of the antecedents of the stress and injury model presented above.

The body of literature has generally supported all three injury antecedent areas as significant predictors of injury, albeit with incredible variance in methodology. Psychosocial factors receiving the most attention that have been consistently tied to injury risk include competitive trait or sport anxiety and life event stress, both of which resulted in vulnerability to injury. Additionally, the presence of coping resources appears to protect against injury risk, whereas the lack of these resources heightens injury risk.

Personality

In their original model, Andersen and Williams (1988) hypothesised that certain positive personality traits (such as hardiness) enabled athletes to view athletic situations as challenging rather than threatening, resulting in a lower stress response and subsequently lower injury risk. Moreover, it was hypothesised that negative personality traits (for example, competitive trait anxiety) will increase stress reactivity. Based on the knowledge available, Andersen and Williams (1988) proposed five specific personality variables that influence stress reactivity: 1) hardiness; 2) locus of control (who or what is responsible for what happens); 3) sense of coherence (a belief that the world is predictable and meaningful); 4) competitive trait anxiety; and 5) achievement motivation (the need to meet goals and experience a sense of achievement).

Across 45 studies in our review examining personality, we documented more than 20 different personality characteristics. Approximately 69 per cent of those studies reported at least some significant relationship between personality and injury outcome. Personality characteristics that have been studied in the stress and injury literature included anger, depression, anxiety (that is, general, competitive/sport anxiety, sport injury anxiety), mood, athletic identity, self-esteem, sport confidence, self-efficacy (both general and physical), physical self-perception, locus of control, mental toughness, optimism, hardiness, motivation (that is, athlete goal orientation), narcissism, neurosis, perceived risk taking, sensation seeking, social desirability, type A (anger, hostility, and so on), exercise dependence, competitiveness and psychological wellbeing. While the breadth of this work is impressive, any synthesis of the work is difficult to draw, as replication studies are rare. Nevertheless, three personality characteristics have received more attention than others in the literature: anxiety, locus of control and mental/emotional states.

Anxiety

Drawing from the literature, anxiety (competitive anxiety in particular) is by far the most frequently examined personality variable seen as affecting injury onset (Blackwell and McCullagh, 1990; Ford, Eklund and Gordon, 2000; Hanson, McCullagh and Tonymon, 1992; Kolt and Kirkby, 1994; Lavallee and Flint, 1996; Petrie, 1993; Sibold, 2004). Competitive anxiety has been defined as an athlete's tendency to perceive competitive situations as threatening and to respond to these situations with heightened anxiety or feelings of fear and tension (Martens, Vealey and Burton, 1990). Athletes exhibiting competitive anxiety might report racing thoughts, an inability to focus, trouble falling asleep the night before competition and inability to eat anything leading up to a competition, among other symptoms. Much of the research appears to suggest that athletes who display increased levels of competitive anxiety are more likely to incur a sport injury.

Locus of control

Locus of control refers to an athlete's perception of who or what is responsible for what happens to them (Kolt and Kirkby, 1996). In our review, nine studies examined locus of control (Dahlhauser and Thomas, 1979; Ekenman, Hassmen, Koivula, Roll and Felliinder-Tsai, 2001; Hanson *et al.*, 1992; Kerr and Minden, 1988; Kolt and Kirkby, 1994; Pargman and Lunt, 1989; Passer and Seese, 1983; Plante and Booth, 1997; Tyler, 1986). However, only two studies found relationships indicating that a higher internal locus of control was associated with a greater number of injuries (Kolt and Kirkby, 1994; Plante and Booth, 1997).

Mental and emotional states

A number of mental and emotional states have also been significantly associated with injury onset (Junge, 2000). Thus far, the most commonly examined mental and emotional states include mood (Amato, 1995; Falkstein, 1999; Galambos, Terry, Moyle, Locke and Lane, 2005; Lavallee and Flint, 1996; Meyers, LeUnes, Elledge and Sterling, 1992; Rozen and de L Horne, 2007; van Mechelen *et al.*, 1996), anger (Dvorak *et al.*, 2000; Plante and Booth, 1997; Thompson and Morris, 1994) and type A (Ekenman *et al.*, 2001; Fields, Delaney and Hinkle, 1990; Schafer and McKenna, 1985). Based on the findings, athletes who report negative mood states (for example, anger) appear to be more likely to become injured (Dvorak *et al.*, 2000; Ekenman *et al.*, 2001; Fields *et al.*, 1990; Schafer and McKenna, 1985; Thompson and Morris, 1994) or sustain more severe injuries (Lavallee and Flint, 1996). Also, athletes with higher negative mood or overall mood disturbances (such as tension, anxiety, depression) appear more likely to become injured (Amato, 1995; Galambos *et al.*, 2005; Lavallee and Flint, 1996; van Mechelen *et al.*, 1996). Yet, desirable mood states have also been positively associated with injury, such as vigour (energy; Rozen and de L Horne, 2007) and low anger (Plante and Booth, 1997).

> One time, I actually looked up in some book the 'psychology' behind an injury and it stated something like, 'Some injuries are the result of having a fear of failure'. It only validated what I knew all along; the stress, anticipation and the exaggerated level of fear I felt for this fantastic opportunity was silly. Over the course of the summer, pain in my right shin was unbearable; no amount of Biofreeze and ice was helping. Soon, pulling my foot up to properly strike a soccer ball was next to impossible. I was in trouble, but I was too afraid to stop training.
>
> (Lyndsie, a female soccer player, speaks about the impact of personality on her injury)

Impact of personality research on injury occurrence: implications for sport medicine professionals

Research identifying an injury-prone personality has not been fruitful thus far but certain personality characteristics do seem to warrant attention. Based on available evidence to date, it seems appropriate for professionals to give special consideration to those athletes exhibiting competitive anxiety, negative mood states and perhaps also patterns of anger/hostility. This literature underscores the importance of getting to know your athletes. It would be important for sport medicine professionals to be mindful observers of athletes entrusted in their care, taking note of individual dispositions (general patterns of behaviour), so as to be in a better position to determine how an athlete's 'personality' may heighten or reduce injury risk as stress ebs and flows (or evolves) over the season.

Stress history

Of the three antecedents in the stress and injury model, stress history continues to be the most commonly examined. In our review, the majority of the studies (49 of a possible 65) measured stress history (comprising major life events, daily hassles and prior injury history; Williams and Andersen, 1998) and, of those, nearly 80 per cent reported significant relationships between stress history and injury.

Major life events

Within stress history, the majority of research has examined significant life- and sport-related stressful events that may predispose an athlete to injury. The evidence supporting a relationship between life event stress and injury is by far the clearest and most consistent. The more life event stress an athlete experiences, the more likely s/he will suffer injury. Williams and Andersen's (1998) paper reported 27 of 30 studies examining life stress and sport injury found some significant relationship. In their updated review (Williams and Andersen, 2007), they reported that 34 of 40 studies had found some association between life event stress and injury. In our own review, 36 of 46 studies reported significant relationships between life event stress and sport injury.

Daily hassles

Daily hassles or minor life events are also considered part of one's stress history. These occur more frequently than major events and thus can also create demands for resources and influence stress reactivity. By definition, daily hassles occur often, yet researchers have not always measured this variable accordingly. It simply may not always be feasible for medical personnel or researchers to take frequent measurements of stress events from athletes, especially while in training. When daily hassles have been measured frequently (weekly or monthly), findings consistently demonstrate significant associations with injury (Byrd, 1993; Fawkner, McMurray and Summers, 1999; Luo, 1994).

Prior injury history

An athlete's injury history (and current injury status) may also contribute to the stress–injury relationship. In one of the few studies to examine multiple stress history factors, van Mechelen *et al.* (1996) found that athletes with a prior injury history were over nine times more likely to become injured than athletes without an injury history. Furthermore, prior injury history was also found to be the strongest predictor of more than 20 different psychological and physical risk factors they examined.

> *In the summer of 2002, I left my NCAA Division II programme to pursue the chal-lenge of a Division I soccer programme. This was extremely anxiety-provoking, but the training schedule was much more intense than I was used to and was over-whelming. I trained very hard all summer, terrified of walking into preseason unprepared and under-trained and basically, failing. This experience was not a challenge; it was a death wish. Why would I leave the cushion and comfort of the Colorado Mountains for the South (which I knew nothing about) and step up a Division? I knew I was becoming complacent in my Division II play, coming in as a freshman and earning a starting spot right away. I was also cranky for selling myself short in the first place and not going Division I to begin with.*
>
> *(Lyndsie, speaks about the impact of prior life event stress on her injury)*

Impact of stress history research on injury occurrence: implications for sport medicine professionals

Existing literature seems to indicate a strong relationship between stress history and sport injury risk. Across three different reviews (Appaneal *et al.*, 2009; Williams and Andersen, 1998, 2007), approximately 80–90 per cent of studies have demonstrated significant associations between stress and sport injury, thus supporting the central role of stress reactivity as underpinning the stress and injury relationship. Therefore, to minimise the possible risks of injury, athletes, coaches and sport medicine profes-sionals should be particularly sensitive to increased stress levels, including both major and minor events, and regardless of whether events are perceived to be posi-tive or negative. Specific ways to monitor stress may include the use of a stress journal or log, or simply ensuring frequent interactions and/or continuous open communication between athletes and their preferred support network (coaches, team physicians, sport psychologists, and so on). Should there be a need to imple-ment systematic programmes for monitoring stress, appropriately trained staff could integrate this into commonly used protocols for monitoring physical training loads and balancing athletes' intensity of effort and rest to maximise performance and avoid overtraining (Kellmann, 2010).

Coping resources

In comparison to personality and stress history antecedents, fewer studies ($n = 31$) have examined athletes' coping resources of which less than 60 per cent reported some significant relationship between coping resources and athletic injury. Inconsistent methodology and lack of replication of research on coping resources make it difficult to extract meaningful findings and to translate them into practical guidelines. For the purposes of this chapter, and to enable us to make sense of the information available, we consider the varied definitions and multifaceted nature of coping resources. Specifically, coping resources in this chapter reflect internal factors such as general coping behaviours (for example, self-care, sleep, nutrition), psychological coping or mental skills (for example, management of thoughts, energy/emotion, attention/focus), as well as external factors (such as social support). Simply stated, coping resources includes an athletes' personal and environmental strengths and vulnerabilities in managing the demands of stress.

Among ten studies that examined stress history and coping resources, seven reported significant findings and five of those reported moderating effects of coping resources (Hardy, Richman and Rosenfeld, 1991; Luo, 1994; Petrie, 1992, 1993; Smith, Smoll and Ptacek, 1990). Among these five studies, stress history accounted for up to 32 per cent of the variance in injury outcome variables when samples were split according to high or low coping resources. Generally, findings suggest that, among athletes with high life stress, those with low social support were most vulnerable to injury, whereas high social support appeared to protect athletes from injury (Hardy et al., 1991; Luo, 1994; Petrie, 1992, 1993). Further, Smith et al. (1990) found that athletes who were most vulnerable to stress-mediated injury were those who were low in both coping skills and social support, reflecting a conjunctive moderating effect. Interestingly, a few of these studies also demonstrated that, among athletes with low stress, those with high social support were likely to be injured, suggesting that social support may enable athletes to take risks and/or achieve elevated arousal, which in turn may increase injury vulnerability. Overall, from what limited research is available, evidence suggests that coping resources may serve to protect some athletes from injury while, for others, they may result in increased injury vulnerability.

> *Before I got injured, I had zero social support. Looking back now, it was the beginning of the end for my parents, they began a bitter three-year divorce battle that summer. It was difficult to socialise with the team, being older than the incoming freshmen and yet still wanting to fit in. Plus, the entire culture was a shock to me, a Midwesterner. I had never experienced anything the South had to offer; the people, the churches, the dry counties.*
>
> *(Lyndsie speaks about a lack of coping resources prior to her injury)*

Impact of coping resource research on injury occurrence: implications for sport medicine professionals

The limited and mixed findings for coping resources merely reinforce the need for sport medicine professionals to get to know individual athletes to better understand his or her own unique coping resources within their own sporting environment. Drawing from social support literature, however, it is clear that having a supportive network can enhance an individual's physical and psychological wellbeing. As such, sport medicine professionals should have an awareness of any athletes who may not have a supportive network around them or who appear to be coping with the demands of personal and athletic life in relative isolation.

Psychological interventions

Of the components of the stress and injury model, the most exciting and promising avenue of research is the usefulness of psychological interventions to prevent athletic injury (Johnson, 2007; Williams and Andersen, 2007), yet it continues to be the least investigated area to date. Only five of the 70 studies we reviewed examined the impact of psychological interventions on injury risk (Johnson, Ekengren and Andersen, 2005; Kerr and Goss, 1996; Kolt, Hume, Smith and Williams, 2004; Maddison and Prapavessis, 2005; Perna, Antoni, Baum, Gordon and Schneiderman, 2003). Three of the five studies demonstrated statistical significance (Johnson *et al.*, 2005; Maddison and Prapavessis, 2005; Perna *et al.*, 2003) and the two studies which did not (Kerr and Goss, 1996; Kolt *et al.*, 2004) likely did not have sufficient power (c.f. Andersen and Stoove, 1998; Williams and Andersen, 2007). Importantly, however, all five intervention studies demonstrated a reduction in injuries, which is noticeably and clinically meaningful.

Each of the five intervention studies were grounded in cognitive behavioural stress management (c.f. Meichenbaum, 1977) principles and involved a series of educational and supportive meeting with athletes. Information was targeted at athletes' cognitive appraisals and stress–response symptoms and included providing skills training for enhanced self-awareness, reducing negative effects of stress and promoting self-regulation or self-control through using psychological coping skills. While psychologically based injury prevention programmes may be limited in number, the evidence is clear. Intervention effects provide strong support for psychological services for athletes to mitigate negative health-related consequences of sport participation (such as reduced injury/illness, time loss due to injury).

Impact of psychological intervention research on injury occurrence: implications for sport medicine professionals

Drawing from the limited research presented above, as well as research on use of psychological interventions in sport performance context, there are number of things that should be considered when designing and delivering effective intervention programmes. These include decisions regarding who is best suited to deliver the programme, when and for how long the programme should be offered and which is the best approach to meet the athlete's needs.

Who is responsible for delivery?

While the provision and evaluation of psycho-educational programmes for athletes' health is certainly warranted, those services should be provided by appropriately trained professionals. Specifically, to best ensure that athletes' psychological information is not misused and that their interests remain protected and respected, such professionals should hold credentials from governing sport psychology organisations, state and/or national regulatory boards for sport psychologists. Thus, professionals who have appropriate credentials are most likely going to work ethically and effectively but, most importantly, know how to do so within a competitive sport environment.

When should the programme be offered and for how long?

Researchers have generally agreed that psychological interventions may be most effective if provided prior to the start of athletes' competitive sport seasons (Kerr and Minden, 1988; Maddison and Prapavessis, 2005). Evidence also indicates that health benefits can be achieved with limited contact over a relatively brief period of time. Perna *et al.* (2003) involved seven sessions over three and a half weeks, Johnson *et al.* (2005) conducted six sessions and two follow-up phone calls, and Maddison and Prapavessis (2005) involved six sessions over a four-week period.

What is the best approach?

There are numerous intervention approaches that may be beneficial to assist athletes in dealing with stressful situations. However, as with any psychological interventions, these should be designed and implemented with an individual athlete in mind to ensure a personalised approach to service delivery. For example, programme content delivered to athletes might reflect a cognitive behavioural approach. Intervention such as stress inoculation training (Meichenbaum and Novaco, 1985), involves three distinct phases: conceptualisation, skill acquisition and application. Several other interventions may be suitable to assist athletes in minimising the risk of sport injury, including (but not limited to): cognitive and somatic-based relaxation strategies (for example, diaphragmatic breathing, progressive muscle relaxation, autogenic training); cognitive interventions (for example, self-talk, visual motor behavioural rehearsal, cognitive restructuring); and other common mental skills for performance excellence (goal setting, attribution and self-confidence). For more details on psychological interventions, see Chapters 5–9.

Conclusion

This chapter has (a) introduced the stress and injury model (Andersen and Williams, 1988; Williams and Andersen, 1998); (b) reviewed the different antecedents associated with athlete's stress response; (c) highlighted the role of stress–response mechanisms in increasing sport injury occurrence; (d) summarised the evidence supporting the use of psychological interventions to prevent sport injuries; and (e) throughout the different sections of the chapter, suggested practical strategies for those wishing to translate this knowledge into professional practice (such as sport/performance psychologists and sport medicine professionals).

Since early work in the 1970s, considerable interest in examining the relationship between psychosocial factors and sport injury has taken place. However, this has not typically occurred in a systematic fashion (Johnson, 2007; Junge, 2000; Petrie and Falkstein, 1998; Williams and Andersen, 2007). As a result, the collective impact of this work remains rather elusive for those not well versed in the psychology of sport injury. Methodological inconsistencies and limited replication may be responsible for disparate findings and ultimately hinder any meaningful application of this work into sport injury prediction and prevention efforts. Nonetheless, it is believed that the clinical and practical implications of this work are rarely doubted and thus are of valuable benefit to athletes' health. Specifically, there are no known adverse health consequences or potential drawbacks to offering psychological interventions to reduce athletes' risk of sport injury. As noted by Williams and Andersen (2007), there have only been positive effects of psychosocial intervention programmes and perhaps such efforts may result in added benefits to sport performance and enjoyment. The field of psychological prediction and prevention of sport injury has an opportunity to guide effective programming for sport medicine professionals. Efforts to promote awareness of psychosocial stress in sport and develop ways to minimise or perhaps even avoid sport injury are important, cost effective, associated with no additive risks and may even enhance the athletes' overall sport experience.

CASE STUDY

MaryEllen has coached a women's soccer team as their head coach for over ten years. The team has been consistently successful for the last five years. The women's soccer team has a long tradition of being nationally ranked and the university has a reputation for producing exceptional world leaders. Over the past three years, MaryEllen and the sport medicine staff have observed a rise in illness and injury complaints. These complaints emerge around the last, and usually most important, four weeks of their competitive season. Students are also taking university exams at this time and it has always been a struggle for members of the team to get exams completed when they are travelling on long road trips during the middle of the week. Sarah, one of the team's co-captains, has shared with MaryEllen that many of her team mates feel constantly tired and are having difficulty staying focused on the field. Sarah, herself, has noticed that it has become more challenging to study for prolonged periods of time these last few days. After meeting with a few of the other athletes, MaryEllen decides to call a meeting with the sport medicine staff to come up with a plan for how they might be able to assist the team in staying healthy and strong through the entire season, both currently and perhaps in the future.

——— **?** ———

1. Briefly describe how psychological antecedents might increase athletes' risk of injury.
2. Identify potential psychosocial factors present among the soccer team and within the sport environment that may be contributing to an increased injury and illness complaints.
3. In addition to psychosocial risks, are there any potential psychosocial strengths among this team which may provide them with resilience to adverse effects of stress? If so, identify and describe what these strengths might be.
4. Suggest two possible psychosocial strategies for reducing injury risk among this team.
5. Identify potential advantages and drawbacks to implementing system-wide (or team) psychosocial interventions for health maintenance and injury prevention.

References

Amato, P. (1995) The effects of life stress and psychosocial moderator variables on injuries and performance in hockey players (PhD Doctoral Thesis). Université de Montreal, Canada. Retrieved from http://proquest.umi.com/pqdweb?did=742175931andFmt=7andclientId=15109andRQT=309andVName=PQD.

Andersen, M. B. and Stoove, M. A. (1998) The sanctity of p<.05 obfuscates good stuff: A comment on Kerr and Goss. *Journal of Applied Sport Psychology*, 10(1), 168–73.

Andersen, M. B. and Williams, J. M. (1988) A model of stress and athletic injury: Prediction and prevention. *Journal of Sport and Exercise Psychology*, 10, 294–306.

Andersen, M. B. and Williams, J. M. (1999) Athletic injury, psychosocial factors, and perceptual changes during stress. *Journal of Sports Sciences*, 17, 735–41.

Appaneal, R., Habif, S., Washington, L. and Granquist, M. D. (2009) A systematic review of research examining psychological factors associated with sport injury risk and prevention. Unpublished manuscript. University of North Carolina at Greensboro, NC.

Bergandi, T. A. and Witting, A. F. (1988) Attentional style as a predictor of athletic injury. *International Journal of Sport Psychology*, 19(3), 226–35.

Blackwell, B. and McCullagh, P. (1990) The relationship of athletic injury to life stress, competitive anxiety and coping resources. *Athletic Training*, 25(1), 25–27.

Bramwell, S. T., Masuda, M., Wagner, N. N. and Holmes, T. H. (1975) Psychosocial factors in athletic injuries: Development and application of the social and athletic readjustment rating scale (SARRS). *Journal of Human Stress*, 1(2), 6–20.

Byrd, B. J. (1993) *The Relationship of History of Stressors, Personality, and Coping Resources, with the Incidence of Athletic Injuries* (Master's thesis). University of Colorado. Boulder, CO.

Centers for Disease Control and Prevention (2002) Nonfatal sports- and recreation-related injuries treated in emergency departments, United States, July 2000–June 2001. *MMWR Morbidity and Mortality Weekly Report*, 23(51), 736–40.

Coddington, R. D. and Troxell, J. R. (1980) The effect of emotional factors on football injury rates: A pilot study. *Journal of Human Stress*, 6(4), 3–5.

Conn, J. M., Annest, J. L. and Gilchrist, J. (2003) Sports and recreation related injury episodes in the US population, 1997–99. *Injury Prevention*, 9(2), 117–23.

Cryan, P. D. and Alles, W. F. (1983) The relationship between stress and college football injuries. *Journal of Sports Medicine and Physical Fitness*, 23(1), 52–8.

Dahlhauser, M. and Thomas, M. B. (1979) Visual disembedding and locus of control as variables associated with high school football injuries. *Perceptual and Motor Skills*, 49(1), 254.

Dvorak, J., Junge, A., Chomiak, J., Graf-Baumann, T., Peterson, L., Rosch, D. and Hodgson, R. (2000) Risk factor analysis for injuries in football players. Possibilities for a prevention program. *American Journal of Sports Medicine*, 28(5 Suppl), S69–74.

Ekenman, I., Hassmen, P., Koivula, N., Roll, C. and Felliinder-Tsai, L. (2001) Stress fractures of the tibia: can personality traits help us detect the injury-prone athlete? *Scandinavian Journal Medicine and Science in Sports*, 11(2), 87–95.

Engebretsen, L. and Bahr, R. (eds) (2009) *Why is Injury Prevention in Sports Important?* Oxford: Wiley-Blackwell.

Falkstein, D. L. (1999) Prediction of athletic injury and postinjury emotional response in collegiate athletes: A prospective study of an NCAA Division I football team. *Dissertation Abstracts International*, 60(09B), 199.

Fawkner, H. J., McMurray, N. E. and Summers, J. (1999) Athletic injury and minor life events: A prospective study. *Journal of Science and Medicine in Sport*, 2, 117–24.

Fields, K. B., Delaney, M. and Hinkle, J. S. (1990) A prospective study of type A behavior and running injuries. *Journal of Family Practice*, 30(4), 425–9.

Ford, I. W., Eklund, R. C. and Gordon, S. (2000) An examination of psychosocial variables moderating the relationship between life stress and injury time-loss among athletes of a high standard. *Journal of Sports Sciences*, 18, 301–13.

Galambos, S., Terry, P., Moyle, G., Locke, S. and Lane, A. (2005) Psychological predictors of injury among elite athletes. *British Journal of Sports Medicine*, 39, 351–4.

Hanson, S. J., McCullagh, P. and Tonymon, P. (1992) The relationship of personality characteristics, life stress, and coping resources to athletic injury. *Journal of Sport and Exercise Psychology*, 14(3) 262–272.

Hardy, C. J., Richman, J. M. and Rosenfeld, L. B. (1991) The role of social support in the life stress/injury relationship. *The Sport Psychologist*, 5, 128–39.

Holmes, T. H. (1970) Psychological screening. Paper presented at the Paper presented at the Football injuries workshop, Washington, DC.

Johnson, U. (2007) Psychosocial antecedents of sport injury, prevention and intervention: An overview of theoretical approaches and empirical findings. *International Journal of Sport and Exercise Psychology*, 5, 352–69.

Johnson, U., Ekengren, J. and Andersen, M. B. (2005) Injury prevention in Sweden: Helping soccer players at risk. *Journal of Sport and Exercise Psychology*, 27, 32–8.

Junge, A. (2000) The influence of psychological factors on sports injuries: Review of the literature. *American Journal of Sports Medicine*, 28(5 Suppl), S10–15.

Kellmann, M. (2010) Preventing overtraining in athletes in high–intensity sports and stress/recovery monitoring. *Scandinavian Journal of Medicine and Science in Sports*, 20(Suppl 2), 95–102.

Kerr, G. A. and Goss, J. (1996) The effects of a stress management program on injuries and stress levels. *Journal of Applied Sport Psychology*, 8(1), 109–17.

Kerr, G. A. and Minden, H. (1988) Psychological factors related to the occurrence of athletic injuries. *Journal of Sport and Exercise Psychology*, 10, 167–73.

Kleinert, J. (2007) Mood state and perceived physical states as short term predictors of sport injuries: Two prospective studies. *International Journal of Sport and Exercise Psychology*, 5, 340–51.

Kolt, G. S. and Kirkby, R. J. (1994) Injury, anxiety, and mood in competitive gymnasts. *Perceptual and Motor Skills*, 78(3), 955–62.

Kolt, G. S. and Kirkby, R. (1996) Injury in Australian female competitive gymnasts: A psychological perspective. *Australian Journal of Physiotherapy*, 42, 121–6.

Kolt, G. S., Hume, P. A., Smith, P. and Williams, M. M. (2004) Effects of a stress-management program on injury and stress of competitive gymnasts. *Perceptual and Motor Skills*, 99(1), 195–207.

Lavallee, D. and Flint, F. (1996) The relationship of stress, competitive anxiety, mood state, and social support to athletic injury. *Journal of Athletic Training*, 31(4), 296–99.

Lazarus, R. S. and Folkman, S. (1984) *Stress, Appraisal, and Coping*. New York: Springer Publishing Company.

Luo, Y. (1994) *The Relationship of Daily Hassles, Major Life Events and Social Support to Athletic Injury in Football* (PhD Doctoral Thesis). University of Minnesota, MN: ProQuest Dissertations and Theses.

Maddison, R. and Prapavessis, H. (2005) A psychological approach to the prediction and prevention of athletic injury. *Journal of Sport and Exercise Psychology*, 27(3), 289–310.

Marshall, S. W. and Guskiewicz, K. M. (2003) Sports and recreational injury: the hidden cost of a healthy lifestyle. *Injury Prevention*, 9(2), 100–2.

Martens, R., Vealey, R. S. and Burton, D. (1990) *Competitive Anxiety in Sport*. Champaign, IL: Human Kinetics.

Meichenbaum, D. (1977) *Cognitive Behavioral Modification: An integrative approach*. New York: Plenum.

Meichenbaum, D. and Novaco, R. (1985) Stress inoculation: A preventative approach. *Issues in Mental Health Nursing*, 7(1–4), 419–35.

Meyers, M. C., LeUnes, A., Elledge, J. R. and Sterling, J. C. (1992) Injury incidence and psychological mood state patterns in collegiate rodeo athletes. *Journal of Sport Behavior*, 15(4), 297–306.

Pargman, D. and Lunt, S. D. (1989) The relationship of self-concept and locus of control to the severity of injury in freshman collegiate football players. *Sports Training, Medicine and Rehabilitation*, 1(3), 203–8.

Passer, M. W. and Seese, M. D. (1983) Life stress and athletic injury: Examination of positive versus negative events and three moderator variables. *Journal of Human Stress*, 9, 11–16.

Perna, F. M., Antoni, M. H., Baum, A., Gordon, P. and Schneiderman, N. (2003) Cognitive behavioral stress management effects on injury and illness among competitive athletes: a randomized clinical trial. *Annals of Behavioral Medicine*, 25(1), 66–73.

Petrie, T. A. (1992) Psychosocial antecedents of athletic injury: the effects of life stress and social support on female collegiate gymnasts. *Behavioral Medicine*, 18(3), 127–38.

Petrie, T. A. (1993) Coping skills, competitive trait anxiety, and playing status: moderating effects on the life stress–injury relationship. *Journal of Sport and Exercise Psychology*, 15(3), 261–74.

Petrie, T. A. and Falkstein, D. L. (1998) Methodological and statistical issues in sport injury prediction research. *Journal of Applied Sport Psychology*, 10(1), 26–45.

Plante, T. G. and Booth, J. (1997) Personality correlates of athletic injuries among elite collegiate baseball players: the role of narcissism, anger and locus of control. *Journal of Human Movement Studies*, 32(4), 47–59.

Rogers, T. J. and Landers, D. M. (2005) Mediating effects of peripheral vision in the life event stress/athletic injury relationship. *Journal of Sport and Exercise Psychology*, 27(3), 271–88.

Rozen, W. M. and de L Horne, D. J. (2007) The association of psychological factors with injury incidence and outcome in the Australian Football League. *Individual Differences Research*, 5(1), 73–80.

Schafer, W. and McKenna, J. (1985) Type A behavior, stress, injury and illness in adult runners. *Stress Medicine*, 1, 245–54.

Sibold, J. S. (2004) A comparison of psychosocial and orthopedic data in predicting days missed due to injury. *Dissertation Abstracts International*, 65(11A), 56.

Smith, R. E., Smoll, F. L. and Ptacek, J. T. (1990) Conjunctive moderator variables in vulnerability and resiliency research: Life stress, social support and coping skills, and adolescent sport injuries. *Journal of Personality and Social Psychology*, 58(2), 360–70.

Thompson, N. J. and Morris, R. D. (1994) Predicting injury risk in adolescent football players: the importance of psychological variables. *Journal of Pediatric Psychology*, 19(4), 415–29.

Tyler, S. J. (1986) The effect of stress due to life change and locus of control on injury/illness among collegiate field hockey players (PhD thesis). University of Maryland College Park, College Park, MD. Retrieved from http://proquest.umi.com/pqdweb?did=751469901 andFmt=7andclientId=15109andRQT=309andVName=PQD

van Mechelen, W., Twisk, J., Molendijk, A., Blom, B., Snel, J. and Kemper, H. C. (1996) Subject-related risk factors for sports injuries: a 1-yr prospective study in young adults. *Medicine and Science in Sports and Exercise*, 28(9), 1171–9.

Williams, J. M. and Andersen, M. B. (1998) Psychosocial antecedents of sport injury: Review and critique of the stress and injury model. *Journal of Applied Sport Psychology*, 10, 5–25.

Williams, J. M. and Andersen, M. B. (2007) Psychosocial antecedents of sport injury and interventions for risk reduction. In G. Tenenbaum and R. Eklund (eds), *Handbook of Sport Psychology*, 3rd edn. Hoboken, NJ: Wiley, pp. 379–403.

Williams, J. M., Tonymon, P. and Wadsworth, W. A. (1986) Relationship of life stress to injury in intercollegiate volleyball. *Journal of Human Stress*, 12(1), 38–43.

3

PSYCHOLOGICAL RESPONSES TO INJURY

A review and critique of existing models

Natalie Walker and Caroline Heaney

Introduction

Anyone who has ever experienced a sport injury, whether it be an athlete who has sustained an injury, a coach of an injured athlete or sport medicine professional treating an injured athlete, will be aware that the occurrence of an injury can have both a physical and psychological effect on the athlete. In addition to the physical effects, sport injury may, for example, lead to feelings of frustration, anxiety, depression, anger or isolation (Johnston and Carroll, 1998). Consideration of the psychological responses to injury is important as they can potentially impact on the athlete's rehabilitation behaviour, the overall rehabilitation outcomes and the subsequent return to training and competition (De Heredia, Munoz and Artaza, 2004). Therefore, understanding the process in which athletes psychologically respond to injuries is of importance. According to Walker, Thatcher and Lavallee (2007), sport medicine professionals should be aware of psychological factors impacting on the injury experience if complete holistic recovery is to occur. Such an understanding is vital in an applied context and can be gained through considering the underpinning psychological theory (Cranney *et al.*, 2009; Thompson, 2000). However, it appears that sport medicine professionals rarely receive adequate training in psychological aspects of sport injuries (for example, Arvinen-Barrow, Penny, Hemmings and Corr, 2010) and these aspects are seldom taught at degree level. For example, Heaney, Green, Roston and Walker (2012) examined the current psychology provision within physiotherapy programmes in UK universities with the intention of exploring the nature and extent of psychology covered in physiotherapy programmes, the delivery and perceived importance of any psychology content and the factors influencing psychology provision. The authors found that 41 per cent of participants indicated that their psychology provision did not contain any theoretical underpinning.

Given the importance of understanding the underlying mechanism and theory of psychological reactions to sport injuries, this chapter outlines existing theoretical models that have been developed to describe and explain psychological responses to sport injury. These models provide a framework to help those interacting with injured athletes (for example, sport medicine professionals) to understand psychological responses to injury and their potential impact. They may also help sport medicine professionals in assisting the injured athlete appropriately to allow for holistic recovery. Specifically, grief-response models (see, for example, Kübler-Ross, 1969), cognitive appraisal models (for example, Brewer, 1994), the integrated model of response to athletic injury and rehabilitation process (Wiese-Bjornstal, Smith, Shaffer and Morrey, 1998) and the biopsychosocial model of sport injury rehabilitation (Brewer, Andersen and Van Raalte, 2002) are introduced to the reader and outlined in detail.

Grief-response models

Grief-response models, or stage models as they are sometimes called, have been taken from other areas of research, such as death and dying (for example, Kübler-Ross, 1969) and applied to sport injury (for example, Mueller and Ryan, 1991). The application of grief-response models to sport injury assumes that injury constitutes a form of loss to the individual (for example, the loss of daily practice routines) and thus the onset of a grieving process. They suggest that an athlete will respond to injury in the same way in which people respond to other significant losses, such as the death of a loved one (Brewer, 1994; Evans and Hardy, 1995). This involves progressing through a series of sequential stages. The number of stages varies from model to model but, in Kübler-Ross's (1969) grief-response model, which is the most commonly applied model in the sport injury psychology literature (Walker *et al.*, 2007), there are five stages: denial, bargaining, anger, depression and acceptance.

There is some support for grief-response models in the sport injury domain (see McDonald and Hardy, 1990; Mueller and Ryan, 1991) and there is evidence to show that sport medicine professionals are aware of 'stage-like' responses to sport injury (Arvinen-Barrow *et al.*, 2010). In their theoretical discussion of response to injury, Mueller and Ryan (1991) offered support for the application of the Kübler-Ross (1969) model of recovery from sport injury. Similarly, Gordon (1986) reviewed the clinical and injury literature and found that there was a typical response to sport injury that is very much like the five-stage Kübler-Ross (1969) model. Furthermore, McDonald and Hardy (1990) supported the grief-like response to sport injury in their research exploring the affective, cognitive and behavioural responses of five university-level injured athletes across a four-week injury period. Despite the vast majority of the literature supporting the grief response in the sport injury domain being somewhat dated, there has been some more contemporary literature identifying that sport injury evokes a grief-like response for injured athletes (Mankad and Gordon, 2010).

> *I've definitely seen evidence of all five of these stages in some of the athletes I've worked with. When an injury first occurs it's quite common for an athlete to under-play or 'deny' the injury to themselves and others. That makes treatment at that stage difficult. Anger can come in when they can no longer deny the injury, owing to the impairment it brings. I certainly have athletes who try and bargain with me about my diagnosis and treatment regime, and depression is fairly common once people start to acknowledge the impact of an injury on their world. Acceptance is, I believe, inevitable although it takes different people different amounts of time to accept, but it's only at that point that you really have the athlete 'on board' in their rehabilitation programme.*
>
> *(Janice, sport medicine professional)*

The application of Kübler-Ross's (1969) model to sport injury is intuitively appealing and can describe the responses of some athletes to sport injury. However, not all research is fully supportive of the predictions of the model. Whilst not accepting the grief-response models in their entirety, several researchers have found partial support for grief-response models (Gordon, Milios and Grove, 1991; Udry, Gould, Bridges and Beck, 1997). For example, Udry *et al.* (1997) when examining psychological responses to season-ending injuries amongst national team skiers, provided only partial support for Kübler-Ross's (1969) grief-response model, as they found no support for the bargaining stage and only minimal support for the denial stage but did support the anger, depression and acceptance stages.

Criticisms of the model include the assumption that the stages are sequential and the failure of the model to account for oscillation between the stages (Brewer, 1994; Evans and Hardy, 1995). There has also been a debate over the mislabelling of the term 'denial', where this is proposed to be a term that should be reserved for noncompliant athletes who, despite education about the nature and severity of their injury, refuse to accept its existence (Udry *et al.*, 1997; Walker *et al.*, 2007). Athletes typically do not deny that an injury exists but tend to downplay its sever-ity and limiting factors and, hence, could be denying the severity and not the injury itself (Pearson and Jones, 1992). Furthermore, the model lacks empirical rigour and is not sport-injury specific (Walker *et al.*, 2007).

Grief-response models fail to account for individual differences in responses to injury (Brewer, 1994; Evans and Hardy, 1995; Harris, 2003; Walker *et al.*, 2007). It seems inflexible to suggest that all injured athletes, regardless of their previous expe-riences and circumstances, will react to injury in the same stereotypical way, progressing through each of the stages in turn. In fact, not all athletes will demon-strate negative psychological responses to injury. It is important to acknowledge that the occurrence of an injury can actually lead to positive as well as negative reactions (Udry *et al.*, 1997; Wrisberg and Fisher, 2004). For example, an athlete who has been experiencing a run of poor performance may welcome the onset of an injury, as it may provide a valid excuse for underperformance. Such an athlete is more likely to experience feelings of relief than the feelings of anger and depression predicted by Kübler-Ross's (1969) model. Equally, an athlete who initially had negative reactions to injury may in time be able to derive positive consequences from the injury experience such as an enhanced perspective, increased motivation or the development of other skills such as coping strategies (Podlog and Eklund, 2006; Udry *et al.*, 1997). Such positive consequences are sometimes referred to as secondary gain (Heil, 1993; Taylor and Taylor, 1997). Owing to a lack of support for discrete emotional reactions to sport injury, research has moved away from investigating grief-response models and has instead focused on examining alternative models not based on the process of grieving. Moreover, research in sport setting has paid very little attention to more contemporary grief-response models, such as the dual process model of coping with bereavement (Stroebe and Schut, 1999), which addresses some of the limitations of the Kübler-Ross's model above and has been widely accepted outside the sport injury context as a means of explaining individual reactions to loss.

- Grief-response models assume that a sport injury constitutes a form of loss and thus requires a process of grieving.
- Grief-response models suggest that all injured athletes will pass through the same stages of grieving in the same order and thus do not allow for individual differences in the injury experience.
- It might be worthwhile for researchers to explore more the application of contemporary models of grief (such as the dual process model of coping with bereavement; Stroebe and Schut, 1999) to describe responses to sport injury.

Cognitive appraisal models

As a result of the limitations of grief-response models, cognitive appraisal models came to be more widely accepted as a means of explaining psychological reactions to injury, since they take individual differences into consideration (Brewer, 1994; Evans and Hardy, 1995; Walker *et al.*, 2007). Similar to the models explaining sport injury occurrence (Williams and Andersen, 1998; for more details see Chapter 2), the roots of cognitive appraisal models are found in theories of stress and coping. According to cognitive appraisal models, emotional and behavioural responses to injury are dictated by the individual's cognitive appraisal or subjective interpretation of their injury (Brewer, 1994; Evans and Hardy, 1995). Importance is therefore placed on how the injury is perceived (cognitively appraised) by the individual rather than on the injury itself. An appraisal is a process through which a potentially stressful situation (sport injury) is assessed and the individual's evaluation of the extent of that stress. These appraisals are proposed to occur in two forms, primary and secondary appraisals (Lazarus, 1991). Primary appraisals involve an assessment of what is at stake taking into account challenge, benefit, threat, harm/loss (Lazarus, 1991), whereas secondary appraisals involve an assessment of the coping options available to manage the demand. This would suggest that two athletes with the same injury could appraise the injury in different ways; for example, one could perceive it as a disaster and the other could perceive it as an opportunity to take a break from intensive training (Udry *et al.*, 1997).

> *I currently have two athletes in my squad with very similar injuries, but their reactions to the injury are poles apart! Athlete A, who is fairly young, is being quite emotional about the injury and is quite down about it and is not so good at attending her rehabilitation appointments. In contrast, athlete B, who is a lot more experienced, is taking being injured in her stride – she is positive about her recovery, and is quite proactive in seeking treatment and doing all of the right things to get better. She never misses a rehabilitation session.*
>
> *(Xavier, coach)*

Cognitive appraisal models consequently tend to have four key components: the stressful situation (the injury), cognitive appraisal, emotional responses and consequences (Kolt, 2003). Our appraisals are believed to influence the way in which we cope with a stressful situation. Brewer (1994) proposed a typical model of cognitive appraisal that can be used to explore and describe psychological responses to injury (Figure 3.1). Personal (for example, dispositional or historical attributes of the individual) and situational (for example, injury-related characteristics, variable aspects of the social and physical environment) factors are proposed to mediate how an athlete appraises their injury (Brewer, 1994). Appraisals are proposed to subsequently affect emotional responses (such as anger, depression) and further influence behavioural responses (like adherence to rehabilitation).

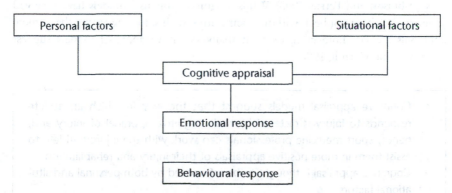

FIGURE 3.1 Typical cognitive appraisal model of psychological adjustment to athletic injury

Source: adapted from Brewer, 1994; reproduced with permission from Taylor & Francis

Given that situational factors impact upon cognitive appraisals, the role of the sport medicine professional and others around the injured athlete should not be underestimated (Wiese-Bjornstal et al., 1998). The sport medicine professional has the capacity to influence the individual's cognitive appraisal of their injury and subsequent emotional reactions and behavioural responses. Walker (2006) identified that the appraisal of the risk of re-injury and the perceived consequences of re-injury caused anxieties about becoming re-injured during rehabilitation and also during re-entry into training and competition in a sample of injured case participants. The athletes stated that re-injury anxieties caused them to be hesitant, cautious and to adopt protective behaviours (such as applying strapping). By using psychological strategies (such as reframing) appraisals can be challenged and adverse responses to athletic injury (like re-injury anxiety) can be reduced (Walker, 2006). Sport medicine professionals might use their understanding of this model to assist an athlete to develop more constructive interpretations of their injury and/or rehabilitation via restructuring to influence more positive emotions and behaviours (for more details on restructuring, see Chapter 8).

Research using cognitive appraisal models in sport injury rehabilitation is considered to be fairly limited (Levy, Polman, Clough and McNaughton, 2006). However, there are studies which support the use of these models. For example, in their study of athletes recovering from knee surgery, Daly, Brewer, Van Raalte, Petitpas and Sklar (1995) found that cognitive appraisal was associated with emotional disturbance, which in turn was inversely related to a measure of adherence. This would suggest that those who cognitively appraise their injury such that it leads to emotional disturbance are less likely to adhere to rehabilitation sessions (Daly et al., 1995) – an important observation for those involved in rehabilitating injured athletes. Similarly, Albinson and Petrie (2003), in their study of 84 US college footballers, reported that they found support for cognitive appraisal models. They found that cognitive appraisal influenced the choice of coping strategy, with those with more negative appraisals tending to adopt more negative coping strategies (Albinson and Petrie, 2003). Whilst cognitive appraisal models have received support, they have not been without their critics, with some suggesting that athlete appraisals are far more complex than many cognitive appraisal models suggest (Johnston and Carroll, 1998).

- Cognitive appraisal models suggest that the way in which an athlete responds to injury is dictated by their cognitive appraisal of injury and, hence, sport medicine professionals can work with the injured athlete to assist them in more positive appraisals of their injury and rehabilitation.
- Cognitive appraisal is thought to be influenced by both personal and situational factors.
- Cognitive appraisal models explain why two athletes may respond to the same injury in different ways.

The integrated model of psychological response to the sport injury and rehabilitation process

Following the development of stage and cognitive appraisal models, Wiese-Bjornstal et al. (1998) proposed that cognitive appraisal and grief-response models are not mutually exclusive. They stated that the sense of loss identified in response to athletic injury is a process that has occurred following a cognitive appraisal and leads to emotions commonly associated with grief (such as depression, anger). They therefore proposed a broader integrated stress-process model, which also subsumes grief as an emotional response; the integrated model of psychological response to the sport injury and rehabilitation process (also known as the integrated model; see Figure 3.2). As well as addressing post-injury factors, this particular model also incorporates pre-injury factors adapted from the model of stress and athletic injury (Andersen and Williams, 1988) discussed in Chapter 2. Wiese-Bjornstal and Smith (1993) reported that the precursors to athletic injury, as outlined in Andersen and Williams' (1988) model, also moderate post-injury responses. For example, high life-stress levels are proposed to not only increase the risk of actual injury but also amplify post-injury mood disturbance. Similarly, Brewer (1994) proposed that the personality traits of hardiness, trait anxiety, extraversion, neuroticism and a pessimistic explanatory style amplified post-injury mood disturbance. It is interesting to note that the modifications to the stress-response model by Williams and Andersen (1998) have not been incorporated into the integrated model (that is, bi-directional arrows between personality, history of stressors, and coping resources; for more details, see Chapter 2).

The remaining sections of Wiese-Bjornstal et al.'s (1998) model extend the theme of the stress response to the post-injury phase, where the injury itself is considered the stressor and the extent of the stress is determined by the athlete's cognitive appraisals, which are influenced by a range of personal and situational factors. The relationship between cognitive appraisal, behavioural response and emotional response is illustrated by the cyclical core of the model (known as the 'dynamic core'). The dynamic core of the model should be viewed as a three-dimensional spiral that heads in an upward direction towards full recovery or in a downward direction away from full recovery if the recovery outcomes (that is, physical and psychosocial outcomes) are negative (Wiese-Bjornstal et al., 1998). The recovery outcomes are centred between the athlete's cognitive appraisal, emotional responses and behavioural responses, implying that all three can directly impact recovery outcomes. The bi-directional arrows in this core represent the dynamic nature of the rehabilitation process. The clockwise arrows indicate that cognitive appraisals affect emotions, which in turn affect behaviour, whilst the anti-clockwise arrows acknowledge that at times the reverse can occur and that changes in direction are possible during rehabilitation (Brewer, 1994; Wiese-Bjornstal et al., 1998). For example, appraisals can affect behaviours, which affect subsequent emotions and appraisals. The dominant process is said to be the appraisals affecting emotions, which subsequently affect behaviours, as seen via the bolder arrows in the dynamic core (Figure 3.3).

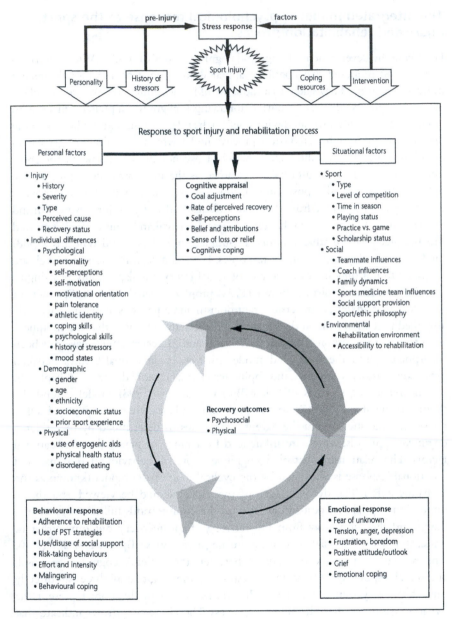

FIGURE 3.2 The integrated model of psychological response to the sport injury and rehabilitation process

Source: adapted from Wiese–Bjornstal *et al.*, 1998; reprinted with permission from Taylor & Francis

> To me, a model like this is really useful, as it helps me to recognise all of the factors that can impact on an athlete's recovery. Before I became aware of this model, I don't think I fully appreciated how influential psychological factors can be on rehabilitation outcomes. I now include psychological assessment and intervention into my work with injured athletes as a matter of course and I often refer athletes to a sport psychologist.
>
> *(Kemal, sport medicine professional)*

The integrated model of psychological response to the sport injury and rehabilitation process is reportedly the most accepted and well-developed model within the sport injury psychology literature (Anderson, White and McKay, 2004; Kolt, 2003; Walker *et al.*, 2007) and, to date, seems to provide the best framework for understanding psychological responses to sport injury. Despite the limited empirical support for the model as a whole, there is some evidence to support some of the individual components of the model. For example, in her in-depth study of the lived experiences of injured athletes, Walker (2006) found support for a range of the personal factors and situational factors identified in the integrated model thought to influence cognitive appraisals. Under 'personal factors' all five injury characteristics listed within the model (history, severity, type, perceived cause, recovery status) were demonstrated, as were the 'individual differences' of personality, pain tolerance, athletic identity, coping skills, history of stressors (Walker, 2006). Under 'situational factors', with the exception of scholarship status, all sport characteristics were evident, as were all of the social mediators. However, she suggested that additional research was needed to determine the similarities and differences in meaning that athletes derive from their lived injury experiences. In an attempt to extend Walker's (2006) study, Grindstaff, Wrisberg and Ross (2010) employed an interview technique based on the philosophical tenets of phenomenology. These authors used a deductive procedure to determine the possible location of the meaning of the injury to each athlete within the framework of the integrated model. Support was offered for a variety of the personal factors (for example, previous injury history, pain tolerance), situational factors (such as playing status, team support), appraisals (for example, uncertainty, knowledge that their present injury state was not permanent), emotions (for example, mild fear of reinjury, trying to stay positive) and behaviours (for example, adherence to rehabilitation) in the model. In contrast, other factors were identified that were not evident within the model (spirituality and religion, belief system, state of the art facilities). Similarly, a wider range of appraisals was identified (for example, believing that the injury is part of God's plan or thinking about the coach's perspective). A broader emotional and behavioural response was also outlined (for example, pleased over timing of injury, surgery anxiety, supporting team mates whilst injured, information gathering, making rehabilitation competitive). Furthermore, whilst support was offered for a range of recovery outcomes evident in the integrated model (for example, discovering meaning in injury) an array of additional recovery outcomes were also discussed (for example, helping team mates to understand the coach's perspective, trusting God) two aspects were outlined as missing from the model: 1) the role of managing medication in the athlete's injury experience; 2) the search for knowledge whilst injured is not limited to the sport medicine professionals (Grindstaff *et al.*, 2010).

Support for the influence of cognitive appraisals on athletes' emotional responses and behavioural responses (the dynamic core of the model) has also been provided by studies that suggest that maintaining a positive outlook has a positive impact on rehabilitation behaviour and recovery (Arvinen-Barrow, Hemmings, Weigand, Becker and Booth, 2007; Heaney, 2006; Tracey, 2003). Walker *et al.* (2007), however critique, the 'dynamic core' of the model and suggest that the relationship between appraisals, emotions, behaviours and recovery outcomes is more complex than the model indicates. As depicted in Figure 3.3. Walker's (2006) results did not lend support for the notion that behavioural responses to injury directly affect subsequent cognitive appraisals and they suggested that this only occurs following an appraisal of the behavioural response. It was also suggested that emotional responses only influence psychosocial recovery outcomes and not physical recovery outcomes. However, physical and psychosocial recovery outcomes were both proposed to be influenced by behavioural responses. The recovery outcomes themselves were also reported to influence subsequent appraisals and appraisals reported to only influence psychosocial recovery outcomes directly (see Walker *et al.*, 2007 for full critique).

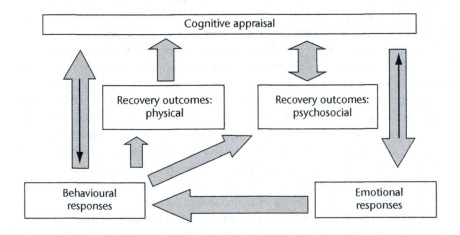

FIGURE 3.3 Critique of the dynamic core of Wiese-Bjornstal *et al.* (1998) integrated model

Source: adapted from Walker *et al.*, 2007; reprinted with permission from Sage Publications

- Wiese-Bjornstal *et al.*'s (1998) model considers both pre-injury and post-injury factors and does not consider grief-response and cognitive appraisal models to be mutually exclusive.
- The model suggests that there is a cyclical relationship between cognitive appraisal of an injury, emotional response to injury and behavioural response to injury that influences, and is influenced by, recovery outcomes.
- The model offers sport medicine professionals a useful framework through which to examine the psychological aspects of sport injury.

A biopsychosocial model of sport injury rehabilitation

One of the main limitations of the integrated model of psychological response to the sport injury and rehabilitation process is that it does not explain how psychological factors influence physical sport injury rehabilitation outcomes (Brewer, 2001; Brewer *et al.*, 2002). Consequently, Brewer *et al.* (2002) proposed the biopsychosocial model of sport injury rehabilitation (Figure 3.4). This model draws upon the approaches increasingly adopted in the healthcare professions, which suggest that health, illness and injury are best understood in terms of an interaction between biological, psychological and social factors, rather than in purely biological terms as is traditional in medicine. Heaney *et al.* (2012) suggest that the biopsychosocial model can have a positive impact on patient satisfaction, empowerment and pain management.

As can be seen in Figure 3.4, the model comprises numerous variables associated with the sport injury rehabilitation process. According to the model, the characteristics of injury and sociodemographic factors influence the biological, psychological and social/contextual factors, which in turn are thought to interact and have an effect on the 'intermediate biopsychological outcomes' such as the pain, rate of recovery and range of motion. The arrow between psychological factors and intermediate biopsychological outcomes is bi-directional, indicating that the biopsychological outcomes can also influence psychological factors. Finally, the model suggests that along with psychological factors, the intermediate biopsychological outcomes affect sport injury rehabilitation outcomes. Again these arrows are both bi-directional indicating that the rehabilitation outcomes can also affect psychological factors and biopsychological outcomes.

I think it's really important to consider an injury and its potential impact from a biopsychosocial perspective. Too many sport medicine professionals look at physiological and psychosocial factors as separate entities when in fact they are undeniably interlinked and interdependent. We're dealing with people and their reactions and so a more holistic approach is required.

(Freda, sport medicine professional)

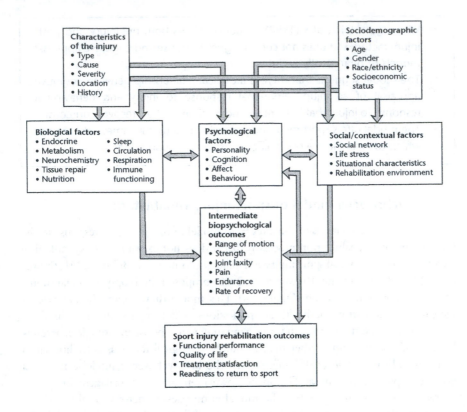

FIGURE 3.4 A biopsychosocial model of sport injury rehabilitation

Source: adapted from Brewer *et al.*, 2002; originally published in D. L. Mostofsky and L. D. Zaichkowsky (eds), *Medical and Psychological Aspects of Sport and Exercise* (2001); reprinted with permission from Fitness Information Technology

A key strength of the model is that it acknowledges that recovery from sport injury occurs in a complex biological, psychological and social matrix and that the interaction of these complex factors is changeable and dynamic (Andersen, 2007). It therefore offers a broad-based framework for understanding responses to sport injury (Brewer, 2001) – one that serves to remind sport medicine professionals of the myriad factors that influence rehabilitation and recovery (Andersen, 2001).

Research directly examining Brewer *et al.*'s (2002) biopsychosocial model of sport injury rehabilitation is sparse; however, there is support available for elements of the model. For example, Brewer (2001) suggested that the correlational relationship seen between emotional reactions to injury and rehabilitation outcomes is consistent with the predictions of the biopsychosocial model. Andersen (2007) has used the 'social/contextual factors' element of the model to examine collaborative relationships during rehabilitation, whilst Andersen (2001) has successfully used the model to examine return to sport participation following injury. Others have provided support more indirectly by advocating a biopsychosocial approach to understanding sport injury, without specifically referencing Brewer *et al.*'s (2002) model (Wiese-Bjornstal, 2009, 2010).

The model does, however, have limitations. Firstly, whilst the model provides explanations for how psychological factors can influence rehabilitation outcomes, it fails to describe the relationships between various psychological factors, particularly in comparison to more psychologically based models (Brewer *et al.*, 2002). Secondly, it has been suggested that, even though the model identifies relevant variables and general relationships, it is not a theory and consequently does not provide a comprehensive explanation as to how different components interact to produce different outcomes (Podlog and Eklund, 2007). Podlog and Eklund (2007) also criticise the model for failing to indicate which factors are most significant in producing various outcomes and why. Heaney *et al.* (2012), in their exploration of current psychology provision within physiotherapy programmes in UK universities, reported that, within the learning outcomes of participant universities' modules and programmes, there is often reference made to the biopsychosocial model but detailed guidance on its interpretation appears to be lacking. Furthermore, there is often a lack of confidence to use a biopsychosocial approach effectively, perhaps owing to inadequacies in training in this area (Green, Jackson and Klaber Moffett, 2008).

Brewer *et al*'s. (2002) model is based on the biopsychosocial approach, which suggests that rehabilitation outcomes are a consequence of a dynamic and complex biological, psychological and social interaction.

Conclusion

The aim of this chapter was to provide a review and critique of the theoretical frameworks of psychological responses to injury to help the sport medicine professional better understand the athlete's injury experiences and factors that might impact their rehabilitation. A range of models have been proposed that seek to describe and explain athlete responses to sport injury each with its own inherent strengths and weaknesses. However, as has been described in this chapter, to date it is Wiese-Bjornstal *et al.*'s (1998) integrated model of psychological response to the sport injury and rehabilitation process that has been acknowledged as the most comprehensive framework.

All of the models have one thing in common – they help to emphasise the importance of psychological responses to the rehabilitation process. This is perhaps the most salient point as, once those around the injured athlete recognise the potential impact of psychological responses, they are more likely to employ interventions aimed at addressing any adverse psychological responses.

CASE STUDY

Gabriella, aged 35, is a Spanish international 400-metre hurdler who has recently sustained an Achilles tendon injury. Gabriella is in the twilight of her international career but has one unfulfilled ambition – to compete in an Olympic Games. Gabriella missed out on selection for the last Olympics owing to injury and realises that, given her age, qualifying for the next Olympics is likely to be her last chance. Consequently, Gabriella has been feeling extremely angry and frustrated about the injury and is anxious to return to full training as soon as possible, to maximise her chances of selection. Before the injury, Gabriella's training had been going extremely well – she has been training with a new coach for a year and her performances had been improving. Gabriella has experienced a similar injury in the past, from which she did recover relatively quickly, but she has been told by her sport medicine professional that because of her age and injury history, her recovery may take a little longer this time. Gabriella feels that this is time that she just doesn't have and she is eager to get a second opinion. The sport medicine professional is concerned that Gabriella is trying to rush her rehabilitation and she will try to return to full training too soon, thus making the injury worse.

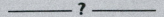

1. Which factors outlined in the case study may affect Gabriella's cognitive appraisal of her injury?
2. What impact might her cognitive appraisal have on her emotional and behavioural responses?
3. Consider how Gabriella's cognitive appraisal of the injury and consequent responses may be different to an athlete sustaining the same injury but at a different stage in their career.

References

Albinson, C. B. and Petrie, T. A. (2003) Cognitive appraisals, stress, and coping: Preinjury and postinjury factors influencing psychological adjustment to sport injury. *Journal of Sport Rehabilitation*, 12, 306–22.

Andersen, M. B. (2001) Returning to action and the prevention of future injury. In J. Crossman (ed.), *Coping with Sports Injuries: Psychological strategies for rehabilitation*. New York: Oxford University Press, pp. 162–73.

Andersen, M. B. (2007) Collaborative relationship in injury rehabilitation: Two case examples. In D. Pargman (ed.), *Psychological Bases of Sport Injuries*, 3rd edn. Morgantown, WV: Fitness Information Technology, pp. 219–236.

Andersen, M. B. and Williams, J. M. (1988) A model of stress and athletic injury: Prediction and prevention. *Journal of Sport and Exercise Psychology*, 10, 294–306.

Anderson, A. G., White, A. and McKay, J. (2004) Athletes' emotional responses to injury. In D. Lavallee, J. Thatcher and M. Jones (eds), *Coping and emotion in sport*. New York: Nova Science, pp. 207–21.

Arvinen-Barrow, M., Hemmings, B., Weigand, D. A., Becker, C. A. and Booth, L. (2007) Views of chartered physiotherapists on the psychological content of their practice: A national follow–up survey in the United Kingdom. *Journal of Sport Rehabilitation*, 16, 111–21.

Arvinen-Barrow, M., Penny, G., Hemmings, B. and Corr, S. (2010) UK chartered physio-therapists' personal experiences in using psychological interventions with injured athletes: An interpretative phenomenological analysis. *Psychology of Sport and Exercise*, 11(1), 58–66.

Brewer, B. W. (1994) Review and critique of models of psychological adjustment to athletic injury. *Journal of Applied Sport Psychology*, 6, 87–100.

Brewer, B. W. (2001) Emotional adjustment to sport injury. In J. Crossman (ed.), *Coping with Sport Injuries: Psychological strategies for rehabilitation*. New York: Oxford University Press, pp. 1–19.

Brewer, B. W., Andersen, M. B. and Van Raalte, J. L. (2002) Psychological aspects of sport injury rehabilitation: Toward a biopsychological approach. In D. I. Mostofsky and L. D. Zaichkowsky (eds), *Medical Aspects of Sport and Exercise*. Morgantown, WV: Fitness Information Technology, pp. 41–54.

Cranney, J., Turnbull, C., Provost, S. C., Martin, F., Katsikitis, M., White, F. A., Voudouris, N. J., Montgomery, I. M., Heaven, P. C. L., Morris, S., Varcin, K. J. (2009) Graduate attrib-utes of the 4–year Australian undergraduate psychology program. *Australian Psychologist*, 44(4), 253–262.

Daly, J. M., Brewer, B. W., Van Raalte, J. L., Petitpas, A. J. and Sklar, J. H. (1995) Cognitive appraisal, emotional adjustment, and adherence to rehabilitation following knee surgery. *Journal of Sport Rehabilitation*, 4(1), 23–30.

De Heredia, R. A. S., Munoz, A. R. and Artaza, J. L. (2004) The Effect of Psychological Response on Recovery of Sport Injury. *Research in Sports Medicine*, 12(1), 15–31.

Evans, L. and Hardy, L. (1995) Sport injury and grief response: A review. *Journal of Sport and Exercise Psychology*, 17, 227–245.

Gordon, S. (1986) Sport psychology and the injured athlete: A cognitive–behavioral approach to injury response and injury rehabilitation. *Sport Science Periodical on Research and Technology in Sport*, March, 1–10.

Gordon, S., Milios, D. and Grove, R. (1991) Psychological aspects of the recovery process from sport injury: The perspective of sport physiotherapists. *Australian Journal of Science and Medicine in Sport*, 23(2), 53–60.

Green, A. J., Jackson, D. A. and Klaber Moffett, J. A. (2008) An observational study of phys-iotherapists' use of cognitive-behavioural principles in the management of patients with back pain and neck pain. *Physiotherapy*, 94(4), 306–13.

Grindstaff, J. S., Wrisberg, C. A. and Ross, J. R. (2010) Collegiate athletes' experience of the meaning of sport injury: A phenomenological investigation. *Perspectives in Public Health*, 130(3), 127–35.

Harris, L. L. (2003) Integrating and analyzing psychosocial and stage theories to challenge the development of the injured collegiate athlete. *Journal of Athletic Training*, 38(1), 75–82.

Heaney, C. (2006) Physiotherapists' perceptions of sport psychology intervention in profes-sional soccer. *International Journal of Sport and Exercise Psychology*, 4(1), 67–80.

Heaney, C., Green, A. J. K., Rostron, C. L. and Walker, N. (2012) A qualitative and quantita-tive investigation of the psychology content of UK physiotherapy education programs. *Journal of Physical Therapy Education*, 26(3), 24–56.

Heil, J. (1993) *Psychology of sport injury.* Champaign, IL: Human Kinetics.

Johnston, L. H. and Carroll, D. (1998) The context of emotional responses to athletic injury: A qualitative analysis. *Journal of Sport Rehabilitation,* 7, 206–20.

Kolt, G. S. (2003) Psychology of injury and rehabilitation. In G. S. Kolt and L. Snyder-Mackler (eds), *Physical Therapies in Sport and Exercise.* London: Churchill Livingstone, pp. 165–83.

Kübler-Ross, E. (1969) *On Death and Dying.* London: MacMillan.

Lazarus, R. S. (1991) *Emotion and Adaptation.* New York: Oxford University Press.

Levy, A. R., Polman, R. C. J., Clough, P. J. and McNaughton, L. R. (2006) Adherence to sport injury rehabilitation programmes: A conceptual review. *Research in Sports Medicine,* 14(2), 149–62.

McDonald, S. A. and Hardy, C. J. (1990) Affective response patterns of the injured athlete: An exploratory analysis. *The Sport Psychologist,* 4, 261–74.

Mankad, A. and Gordon, S. (2010) Psycholinguistic changes in athletes' grief response to injury after written emotional disclosure. *Journal of Sport Rehabilitation,* 19(3), 328–42.

Mueller, F. O. and Ryan, A. (eds) (1991) *The Sports Medicine Team and Athletic Injury Prevention.* Philadelphia, PA: Davis.

Pearson, L. and Jones, G. (1992) Emotional effects of sports injuries: Implications for physiotherapists. *Physiotherapy,* 78(10), 762–70.

Podlog, L. and Eklund, R. C. (2006) A Longitudinal Investigation of Competitive Athletes' Return to Sport Following Serious Injury. *Journal of Applied Sport Psychology,* 18(1), 44–68.

Podlog, L. and Eklund, R. C. (2007) Psychosocial considerations of the return to sport following injury. In D. Pargman (ed.), *Psychological bases of sport injuries,* 3rd edn. Morgantown, WV: Fitness Information Technology, pp. 109–30.

Stroebe, M. S. and Schut, H. (1999) The dual process model of coping with bereavement: Rationale and description. *Death Studies,* 23, 197–224.

Taylor, J. and Taylor, S. (1997) *Psychological Approaches to Sports Injury Rehabilitation.* Gaithersburg, MD: Aspen.

Thompson, N. (2000) *Theory and Practice in Human Services.* Buckingham: Open University Press.

Tracey, J. (2003) The emotional response to the injury and rehabilitation process. *Journal of Applied Sport Psychology,* 15(4), 279–93.

Udry, E., Gould, D., Bridges, D. and Beck, L. (1997) Down but not out: Athlete responses to season-ending injuries. *Journal of Sport and Exercise Psychology,* 19, 229–48.

Walker, N. (2006) The meaning of sports injury and re-injury anxiety assessment and intervention (PhD dissertation). University of Wales, Aberystwyth.

Walker, N., Thatcher, J. and Lavallee, D. (2007) Psychological responses to injury in competitive sport: A critical review. *Journal of The Royal Society for the Promotion of Health,* 127(4), 174–80.

Wiese-Bjornstal, D. M. (2009) Sport injury and college athlete health across the lifespan. *Journal of Intercollegiate Sport,* 2(1), 64–80.

Wiese-Bjornstal, D. M. (2010) Psychology and socioculture affect injury risk, response, and recovery in high-intensity athletes: a consensus statement. *Scandinavian Journal of Medicine and Science in Sports,* 20, 103–11.

Wiese-Bjornstal, D. M. and Smith, A. M. (1993) Counseling strategies for enhanced recovery of injured athletes within a team approach. In D. Pargman (ed.), *Psychological bases of sport injuries.* Morgantown, WV: Fitness Information Technology, pp. 149–82.

Wiese-Bjornstal, D. M., Smith, A. M., Shaffer, S. M. and Morrey, M. A. (1998) An integrated model of response to sport injury: Psychological and sociological dynamics. *Journal of Applied Sport Psychology,* 10, 46–69.

Williams, J. M. and Andersen, M. B. (1998) Psychosocial antecedents of sport injury: Review and critique of the stress and injury model. *Journal of Applied Sport Psychology*, 10, 5–25.

Wrisberg, C. A. and Fisher, L. A. (2004) The benefits of injury. *Athletic Therapy Today*, 9(6), 50–1.

4

PSYCHOLOGICAL ASPECTS OF REHABILITATION ADHERENCE

Megan D. Granquist and Britton W. Brewer

Introduction

Existing theoretical frameworks (for more details, see Chapter 3) and empirical evidence are in agreement that rehabilitation adherence is an essential component for successful sport injury rehabilitation (Arnheim and Prentice, 2000; Bassett, 2003; Bassett and Prapavessis, 2007; Fisher, Mullins and Frye, 1993; Flint, 1998; Kolt, Brewer, Pizzari, Schoo and Garrett, 2007; Taylor and May, 1996; Udry, 1997). More specifically, rehabilitation nonadherence has been associated with poorer overall rehabilitation outcomes (for example, functional ability, strength, range of motion; (Brewer, 1998; Brewer *et al.*, 2000) and potentially has an impact on increasing the risk of re-injury (Arnheim and Prentice, 2000).

Despite the importance of adherence for physical and psychological recovery, suboptimal sport injury rehabilitation adherence rates of patients have been found for clinics working with sport injuries. For example, in a study by Taylor and May (1996), 60 per cent of patients reported that they were not fully adherent with prescribed home modalities (such as cryotherapy) and 54 per cent reported that they were not fully adherent with prescribed rest. Udry (1997) reported adherence at 79 per cent for athletes receiving physical therapy following anterior cruciate ligament reconstruction, with highest rates at the beginning of rehabilitation. In a review of the literature, Brewer (1998) reported adherence rates ranging from 40–91 per cent.

One of the ways in which rehabilitation adherence can be improved is through the use of psychological interventions (see, for example, Garza and Feltz, 1998). Existing literature, albeit limited, has suggested that comprehensive psychological skills training programmes that include goal setting, stress management techniques and a range of coping strategies may be transferable to the rehabilitation setting with the aim of improving adherence. Given the importance of adherence in sport injury rehabilitation, this chapter outlines the psychological aspects of sport injury rehabilitation adherence. More specifically, the chapter (a) defines adherence; (b) provides a theoretical basis to rehabilitation adherence; (c) highlights the importance of rehabilitation adherence/nonadherence; (d) provides an outline of the role of psychological interventions in facilitating rehabilitation adherence; (e) discusses the role of sport medicine professionals in facilitating adherence; and (f) introduces different ways in which adherence could be measured.

Rehabilitation adherence: conceptual clarity

When defining adherence, researchers across discipline boundaries appear to be in agreement of what it entails. However, there are inconsistencies in defining adherence. An accepted definition of adherence among professionals who use exercise as rehabilitation from disease is 'an active, voluntary collaborative involvement of the patient in a mutually acceptable course of behaviour to produce a desired preventative or therapeutic result' (Meichenbaum and Turk, 1987: 20). The above definition can also be beneficial in the sport injury rehabilitation context. Similar to exercise prescribed for a specific medical condition or disability to facilitate recovery from a condition (such as heart attack or knee injury), the driving motivation for sport injury rehabilitation is to return back to a pre-injury level of ability and fitness. In general medicine and health, adherence has been defined as 'the degree to which patient behaviours coincide with the recommendations of health-care providers' (Vitolins, Rand, Rapp, Ribisl and Sevick, 2000: 188S). These definitions both highlight the importance of the patient's voluntary action in following professional recommendations.

Within the broader areas of exercise psychology and behavioural medicine, '[a]dherence refers to maintaining an exercise regimen for a prolonged period of time... Central to adherence is the assumption that the individual voluntarily and independently chooses to engage in the activity' (Lox, Martin Ginis and Petruzzello, 2006: 6–7). This definition of exercise adherence is in line with the medical and health areas and can be applied to sport injury rehabilitation. In both exercise and injury rehabilitation contexts, the desired behaviours must be maintained for a period of time. However, while exercise adherence behaviour may be motivated by long-term health promotion, in the sport rehabilitation context there is arguably an immediate motivating component (for example, recovery from injury, return to competitive sport, return to play pressures). Similar to exercise adherence, rehabilitation adherence also relies on an individual choosing to engage in the rehabilitation and to what degree. However, exercise adherence applies to behaviour to be maintained continuously over the lifespan, whereas rehabilitation is a time-limited set of behaviours aimed at returning to normal function.

It appears that the terms adherence and compliance have been often used interchangeably (Bassett and Prapavessis, 2007; Taylor and May, 1996). The term adherence is typically associated as a description of a behaviour that is aimed at a particular outcome, whereas compliance can be defined as an individual's willingness to follow and engage in the required behaviours. Thus, in the context of this chapter, sport injury rehabilitation adherence is seen as the extent to which an individual completes behaviours as part of a treatment regimen designed to facilitate recovery from injury.

Rehabilitation adherence: theoretical basis

Theoretical models serve as frameworks for understanding the rehabilitation process and for guiding research. Understanding psychological models of sport injury are useful because they provide a conceptual overview from which the antecedents and outcomes of rehabilitation adherence can be investigated. Thus far, a number of theoretical approaches have been found useful in understanding rehabilitation adherence (Brewer, 1998), of which the rehabilitation schematic (Brewer et al., 2000) will be introduced first as it shows the mediating and moderating roles of adherence in sport injury rehabilitation, followed by a biopsychosocial model of sport injury rehabilitation (Brewer, Andersen and Van Raalte, 2002). These two models are seen as useful to sport medicine professionals, sport psychology consultants and other professionals interested and involved in conceptualising rehabilitation adherence in the context of both psychological and physical rehabilitation and recovery.

Rehabilitation schematic: the role of adherence

Several theoretical frameworks (for example, Wiese-Bjornstal, Smith, Shaffer and Morrey, 1998) have proposed that a person's cognitive appraisals of and emotional responses to the injury are seen as factors influencing behaviour during rehabilitation. These models also propose that cognitive appraisals, emotional and behavioural responses are all influenced by a number of personal and situational factors. The interaction between individuals' cognitive appraisals, emotional responses and behavioural responses is thought to have an impact on the rehabilitation process and overall physical and psychological outcomes. Brewer et al. (2000) proposed that rehabilitation adherence as a behavioural response can also mediate the relationship between psychological factors and rehabilitation outcomes. According to Brewer and colleagues, rehabilitation adherence can act as a mediator between psychological factors and rehabilitation outcomes, thus highlighting the importance of adherence as part of successful rehabilitation (Figure 4.1).

The biopsychosocial model of sport injury rehabilitation

In general medicine and health, as well as in sport injury rehabilitation, physical factors (for example, type and severity of injury, health status of patient) affect overall recovery following an injury; however, more recently, psychological and social factors have also received attention as contributors to recovery. The biopsychosocial model of sport injury rehabilitation can serve as a guide for sport injury rehabilitation professionals by providing an inclusive framework from which physical, psychological and social factors influencing the sport injury rehabilitation

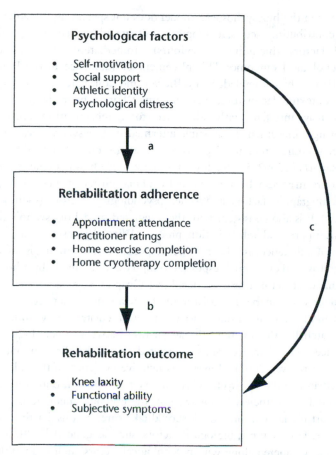

FIGURE 4.1   Schematic representation of hypothesised relationships among psychological factors, rehabilitation adherence and rehabilitation outcome

Source: adapted from Brewer *et al.*, 2000; reprinted with permission from the American Psychological Association

process and outcomes can be better understood (Brewer, Andersen, *et al.*, 2002). As discussed in Chapter 3, the biopsychosocial model provides a conceptual framework that ties biological, psychological and social factors to rehabilitation outcomes. This model acknowledges injury characteristics and socio-demographic factors as influencing biological factors, psychological factors and social/contextual factors. The model proposes that biological, psychological, and social/contextual factors are interrelated and reciprocally affect intermediate biopsychological responses, which, in turn, are proposed to directly influence sport injury rehabilitation outcomes. In other words, adherence, as a behavioural response to sport injury, can have an impact on an individual's range of motion, strength, joint laxity, pain, endurance and rate of recovery (Brewer, Andersen, *et al.*, 2002).

Although the biopsychosocial model does not specifically list adherence as one of the contributing factors, it is logical to situate adherence, among other psychological factors (including behaviours), immediately prior to intermediate biopsychological outcomes. This placement of adherence in the biopsychosocial model is clearly acknowledged by Brewer and colleagues when describing how social/contextual factors influence outcomes: 'For example, disruptive life circumstances may interfere with adherence to a rehabilitation protocol, thereby hampering achievement of favorable intermediate biopsychological outcomes and, ultimately, desired functional performance at the end of rehabilitation' (Brewer, Andersen, *et al.*, 2002: 50). Such would imply a nice fit for adherence because these behaviours may also be influenced by injury characteristics, biological factors, sociodemographic factors and other psychological factors (such as cognition, emotion). It is also consistent with the integrated model of psychological response to sport injury and rehabilitation process (Wiese-Bjornstal *et al.*, 1998), which holds that adherence, as a behavioural response to sport injury, is affected directly by cognitive and emotional responses to injury and indirectly by a host of personal and situational factors (for more details, see Chapter 3). As such, it can be suggested that adherence can be a mediator of the relationship between biopsychosocial factors and rehabilitation outcomes (both intermediate and overall).

Research has documented the association between psychological factors and adherence and adherence being correlated with rehabilitation outcomes (for a review, see Brewer, 2007). However, conclusive evidence of the role of adherence as a mediator of the biopsychosocial factors–rehabilitation outcome relationship is still limited. Nevertheless, being aware of the potential mediational role of adherence, sport medicine professionals should take care to consider the antecedents to adherence. For example, biological factors, such as general health and nutrition, should be considered along with psychological factors, such as an athlete's personality, mood, cognition and behaviour, and social factors, such as status within the team and family situation. Using the biopsychosocial model of sport injury rehabilitation (Brewer, Andersen, *et al.*, 2002) as a framework for treating injured athletes, can help sport medicine professionals to adopt a holistic approach to rehabilitation and thus help them recognise aspects influencing adherence beyond the more-obvious biological factors.

> Understanding the theoretical basis of rehabilitation adherence sets a framework from which sport medicine professionals can conceptualise adherence antecedents and resultant behaviours.

The impact of rehabilitation nonadherence

Although researchers and sport medicine professionals commonly agree that rehabilitation adherence is useful to achieve successful recovery from a sport-related injury, many questions remain to be answered surrounding the role of rehabilitation adherence in overall recovery outcomes. Indeed, research on the relationship between rehabilitation adherence and rehabilitation outcomes in the sport injury domain has produced mixed findings, with multiple examples of positive, nonsignificant and negative adherence–outcome associations (for a review, see Brewer, 2007). If the adherence–outcome relationship for a given rehabilitation programme is nonsignificant or positive, nonadherence to rehabilitation is unlikely to be harmful (and might even be helpful). When the appropriate level of rehabilitation activities required to achieve desired rehabilitation outcomes is known (for example, Bohannon *et al.*, 2008; Boyce and Brosky, 2008; Ryan *et al.*, 2009), nonadherence can be risky or harmful. For example, doing fewer rehabilitation activities than prescribed might slow recovery, whereas overdoing rehabilitation activities might result in re-injury or injury to another part of the body. To date, the appropriate dose of adherence remains unknown; it is important to call for further research. Identifying dose–response relationships for commonly prescribed rehabilitation protocols would be of importance, as such inquiry could provide an answer to the clinically important question of 'to what degree do athletes need to adhere to their rehabilitation protocols to achieve optimal rehabilitation outcomes?' This information would be useful to sport medicine professionals in guiding their expectations for athletes' rehabilitation behaviours and subsequently affecting overall rehabilitation outcomes. Nevertheless, in the absence of such information, it is important to monitor and measure adherence. By doing so, those working with injured athletes can get a clear picture of the rehabilitation process as a whole (including personal and situational factors) and thus plan their treatment more effectively. Moreover, facilitating optimal levels of adherence for each individual athlete can be enhanced through the use of psychological interventions, which when combined with physical rehabilitation can have an effect on adherence and subsequently to rehabilitation outcomes.

> *I think adherence to the athlete's rehab starts with the athletic trainer and making sure the athlete knows what is expected of them from the beginning. I have very few athletes that have poor adherence to rehab. I make it a point to have a good relationship with them and communicate well with them throughout the rehab process. I am fortunate because I have the coach's support. If athletes miss rehab sessions or are not putting forth the effort, then they are talked to by the coach and I've noticed that the athletes' behaviors improve. There are some athletes that I have to watch and really stay on top of them to make sure that they are not doing too much. But, again if I have a good relationship with them then simply communicating with them and explaining the rehab process helps immensely.*
> *(Athletic trainer working at a Division I university in the*
> *National Collegiate Athletic Association, USA)*

Rehabilitation adherence: the role of psychological interventions

Given the potential key role of adherence in achieving desired rehabilitation outcomes, it would seem important to be able to foster athletes' adherence to injury rehabilitation programmes shown to have a beneficial impact on rehabilitation outcomes. The literature on empirically supported treatments to boost adherence to sport injury rehabilitation, however, is extremely limited, consisting of a few studies in which goal setting interventions were applied successfully to enhance adherence (Evans and Hardy, 2002a; Penpraze and Mutrie, 1999). Fortunately, it is possible to draw upon findings from research on predictors of adherence to sport injury rehabilitation and enhancement of adherence to rehabilitation of medical conditions other than sport injury for guidance. In a synthesis of research on factors associated with adherence to rehabilitation, Brewer (2004: 44) concluded that athletes and other clients undergoing rehabilitation are most likely to adhere when they:

- possess personal characteristics that facilitate adhering with a potentially challenging rehabilitation programme (such as self-motivation, tough mindedness);
- experience an environment conducive to adherence (for example, social support for rehabilitation, comfortable and convenient clinical setting);
- perceive their medical condition as sufficiently serious to engender concern but are not overly hampered by pain or emotional distress;
- attribute their health to behaviours within their own control; and
- believe in the efficacy of their rehabilitation programme and are confident in their ability to complete the programme.

In the general rehabilitation literature, educational approaches have been the predominant mode of attempting to enhance adherence. A meta-analysis of patient education interventions for people with back pain indicated a beneficial effect on adherence (DiFabio, 1995). Educational features that have been found to improve the adherence-enhancing impact of rehabilitative interventions include supervision of therapeutic exercises, oversight of rehabilitation by professionals with advanced condition-specific training and augmentation of traditional instructional methods with use of instructional media, such as audio recordings and booklets, with written and illustrated instructions for home exercise activities (for a review, see Brewer, 2004).

Augmented by correlational research (Scherzer et al., 2001) indicating that use of goal setting is positively associated with sport injury rehabilitation adherence, there is experimental evidence (Evans and Hardy, 2002a; Penpraze and Mutrie, 1999) that goal setting can enhance adherence to sport injury rehabilitation programmes. Consistent with the list of circumstances correlated with favourable levels of adherence, goal setting appears to be effective by increasing rehabilitation self-efficacy, attention to the rehabilitation protocol and attribution of recovery to personally controllable factors (Evans and Hardy, 2002b).

A variety of other interventions has been advocated for the enhancement of adherence to sport injury rehabilitation but these interventions lack experimental support for their use. Correlational findings suggest that the use of positive self-talk (Scherzer *et al.*, 2001) and provision of social support (Byerly, Worrell, Gahimer and Domholdt, 1994; Duda, Smart and Tappe, 1989; Fisher, Domm and Wuest, 1988; Johnston and Carroll, 2000) might have a favourable effect on sport injury rehabilitation adherence. In the general rehabilitation literature, multimodal interventions that combine multiple techniques into a single treatment approach have shown potential as a means of enhancing adherence to rehabilitation. For example, a motivationally focused intervention that combined information/counselling, reinforcement of desired rehabilitation behaviour, behavioural contracting and self-monitoring of rehabilitation exercise behaviour achieved short-term gains in physiotherapy attendance for people with low back pain (Friedrich, Gittler, Halberstadt, Cermak and Heiller, 1998). Similarly, combining behavioural contracting, cued recall of the rehabilitation programme, education, goal setting, homework, mental practice of rehabilitation activities and modelling had a beneficial impact on adherence to a rheumatoid arthritis joint protection programme (Hammond and Freeman, 2001).

> Practical issues related to rehabilitation adherence, including psychological and psychosocial intervention strategies, should be considered by sport medicine professionals.

Role of sport medicine professionals in facilitating adherence

Although several personal characteristics of the athlete are correlated with sport injury rehabilitation adherence, these factors are not readily manipulated. Nevertheless, knowledge of the extent to which athletes are self-motivated and tolerant of pain can be used by sport medicine professionals to guide their interactions with athletes and to tailor the rehabilitation regimens that they design to the personal strengths and weaknesses of the athletes. Sport medicine professionals can directly influence adherence behaviour through their use of several common intervention approaches, including education, goal setting, multimodal intervention and communication.

Sport medicine professionals can exert a positive influence on the adherence of the athletes with whom they are working by developing a positive rapport and by simply communicating effectively. Listening to athletes, explaining rehabilitation activities clearly, avoiding jargon and overly technical terminology, controlling nonverbal behaviour, and recognising athletes' needs for informational as well as socio-emotional communication are some ways that sport medicine professionals can interact with athletes to create an environment that is conducive to adherence to rehabilitation.

The injury and year of physical therapy took place when I was 16 and 17. Without physical therapy I wouldn't have the use of my arm. Though it seemed I had so far to go when I first began and I was so frustrated by the pain that I wanted to quit, I look back now and am so grateful for my therapist and the work I did. It even opened a whole new area of academic interest for me and inspired me to major in biology... From a mental standpoint, having a regimented rehabilitation programme and having to go to therapy each day was like a form of training. The only thing I wish was that I had more of a support group of people my own age or of athletes who were also involved in therapy, I felt a bit isolated. My therapist kept me motivated by providing performance-based goals and having high expectations that I had to work hard to meet.
(A former gymnast reflecting on rehabilitation following surgery for complications from a dislocated elbow)

Measuring rehabilitation adherence

Given the importance of facilitating rehabilitation adherence, a number of researchers have used a range of methods to measure adherence. These include attendance at rehabilitation sessions, home exercise completion, compliance with activity restrictions, healing rate and sport medicine professional reports. Attendance at rehabilitation sessions is an objective, easily obtained measure of adherence. Many studies have used attendance either on its own or in conjunction with other adherence measures (Bassett and Prapavessis, 2007; Brewer *et al.*, 2003; Brewer *et al.*, 2000; Daly, Brewer, Van Raalte, Petitpas and Sklar, 1995; Scherzer *et al.*, 2001; Udry, 1997). Home exercise completion has been measured with retrospective self-report questionnaires, daily exercises logs (Bassett and Prapavessis, 2007; Brewer *et al.*, 2003; Brewer *et al.*, 2000; Scherzer *et al.*, 2001; Taylor and May, 1996) and electronic monitoring devices (see, for example, Belanger and Noel, 1990; Levitt, Deisinger, wall, Ford and Cassisi, 1995). Completion of home cryotherapy (that is, icing) has also been collected via self-report measures (Bassett and Prapavessis, 2007; Brewer *et al.*, 2003; Brewer *et al.*, 2000; Scherzer *et al.*, 2001; Taylor and May, 1996). Patient self-report of compliance with activity restrictions (Bassett and Prapavessis, 2007; Taylor and May, 1996) and compliance with strapping/bracing and compliance with elevation (Bassett and Prapavessis, 2007) have also been used to measure sport injury rehabilitation adherence. Some studies have also used healing rate as a measure; however, such can be viewed as totally inappropriate for assessing adherence because it corresponds to a treatment outcome, not to the behavioural process (that is, adherence) that underlies it (Brewer, 1998).

In addition to the above, sport medicine professional's reports have been used regularly in rehabilitation adherence research. For example, Taylor and May (1996) had physiotherapists estimate patients' compliance with home-based rehabilitation protocol (such as mobility, stretching and strengthening exercises, hot/cold therapy, application of compression). Such estimates are unlikely to be any more accurate than patient self-report and, indeed, may be less accurate because the sport medicine professionals are not present when the rehabilitation activities are carried out. However, sport medicine professional ratings of patients' behaviour in clinical settings are wholly appropriate, as the professionals are able to directly observe the behaviour taking place. Several instruments have been developed to record sport medicine professionals' observations of athletes' rehabilitation behaviour in clinical settings, including the sports medicine observation code (Crossman and Roch, 1991), the sport injury rehabilitation adherence scale (SIRAS; Brewer et al., 2000), and the rehabilitation adherence measure for athletic training (RAdMAT; Granquist, Gill and Appaneal, 2010). For the purposes of this chapter, both the SIRAS and the RAdMAT are discussed and presented in more detail.

The sport injury rehabilitation adherence scale (SIRAS)

The SIRAS is a widely used measure of adherence to clinic-based activities. It has demonstrated strong psychometric properties and has been used in research with rehabilitation clinics (see, for example, Bassett and Prapavessis, 2007; Brewer et al., 2003; Brewer et al., 2000; Daly et al., 1995; Kolt et al., 2007; Scherzer et al., 2001). The SIRAS was developed by the authors from existing literature on adherence. It is a brief measure consisting of three items that ask the sport medicine professional to rate: (1) the patient's intensity of rehabilitation completion; (2) frequency of following instructions and advice; and (3) their receptivity to changes in rehabilitation on a five-point Likert-type scale (range 3–15, with higher scores indicating greater adherence). The instructions of the SIRAS can be modified to refer to a single rehabilitation session or to multiple rehabilitation sessions over a period of time. Research in clinical and clinical analogue settings in Australia, New Zealand and the United States (Brewer, Avondoglio, et al., 2002; Kolt et al., 2007) has yielded high levels of interrater agreement for the SIRAS and shown the ability of the SIRAS to discriminate among low, moderate and high levels of adherence to clinic-based rehabilitation activities.

The rehabilitation adherence measure for athletic training (RAdMAT)

The RAdMAT contains 16 items with ratings on a four-point Likert-type scale (range 16–64, with higher scores indicating greater adherence) with three subscales: (a) attendance/participation (subscale range 5–20); (b) communication (subscale range 3–12); and (c) attitude/effort (subscale range 8–32). Some of the items in the attendance/participation subscale include, 'arrives at rehabilitation on time' and 'follows the prescribed rehabilitation plan'. Items in the communication subscale include, 'communicates with the athletic trainer if there is a problem with the exercises' and 'provides the athletic trainer feedback about the rehabilitation program'. Items in the attitude/effort subscale include, 'gives 100 per cent effort in rehabilitation sessions' and 'is self-motivated in rehabilitation sessions'. Although the RAdMAT was developed for use within athletic training sports medicine settings, the items on the RAdMAT are not specific to the athletic training context and thus may be useful in other sport rehabilitation (such as physiotherapy, sports therapy) settings. The RAdMAT differentiates between the most, average and least adherent athlete, providing evidence for its validity. Furthermore, total scores and subscales for the most, average and least adherent athletes were significantly related to the SIRAS. Both the SIRAS and RAdMAT discriminate among the most, average, and least adherent athletes. With its three subscales, the RAdMAT may be useful for guiding practice and interventions aimed at enhancing rehabilitation adherence. Low ratings on any one of the three subscales might inform intervention efforts during rehabilitation. For example, if a patient rates low on the communication subscale, physiotherapists and/or sport psychology consultants working with the patient might introduce skills to enhance communication.

Conclusion

This chapter has provided the reader with an overview of the psychological aspects of sport injury rehabilitation adherence. First, the concept definitions of adherence were discussed, followed by theoretical explanations of rehabilitation adherence. This was followed by a section highlighting the importance of rehabilitation adherence/nonadherence and a description of the proposed role of psychological interventions in facilitating rehabilitation adherence. The role of sport medicine professionals in facilitating adherence was introduced to the reader and examples of how to measure adherence in a sport injury rehabilitation context were presented. Drawing from the existing literature, it is clear that athlete behaviour in the form of adherence to rehabilitation regimens is a prominent psychological aspect of sport injury rehabilitation. Although adherence is thought to contribute to rehabilitation outcomes, nonadherence is a common problem for clinic-based and, especially, home-based rehabilitation activities. Personal and situational or environmental factors associated with sport injury rehabilitation adherence have been identified and can inform the implementation of adherence enhancement interventions such as education, goal setting and effective sport medicine professional communication. Adherence can be measured in both subjective and objective ways depending on the specific behavioural requirements of the rehabilitation programme in question.

CASE STUDY

Michael is a 22-year old collegiate baseball pitcher attending college approximately 1,500 miles away from home. He comes from a middle-class family in a mid-western state in the United States and his athletic goal is to play baseball in a minor league following college, with the hopes of having a professional baseball career. Last year, Michael's junior year, he sprained the ulnar collateral ligament in his elbow and had subsequent surgery to repair the ligament. Michael has successfully overcome previous injuries but this surgery is his first.

Now, four months following the reconstructive surgery, despite his lack of pain, rehabilitation protocols specify limited activity to limit stresses on the elbow and allow proper tissue healing. Michael is frustrated at his restricted activity (such as limited throw distance, limited throw intensity and limited pitch count). As an athlete, Michael has learned to push his body until he is fatigued or experiencing pain; it is difficult for him to accept that he cannot push himself in rehabilitation as he would on the playing field. Michael is also concerned about his minor league recruitment possibilities because he is not able to demonstrate his pitching skill while he is sidelined. Fortunately, Michael has confidence in and good rapport with the sports medicine professional that is leading his rehabilitation. However, he has considered incorporating additional self-guided throwing exercises to supplement his rehabilitation.

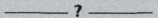

──────── **?** ────────

1. Consider the biopsychosocial model of rehabilitation. In addition to biological factors and injury characteristics, list specific sociodemographic, psychological and social/contextual factors that may influence the sport injury rehabilitation process for Michael.
2. Describe a multimodal intervention that could serve to keep Michael motivated towards his rehabilitation and target rehabilitation adherence. Michael is frustrated at his restricted activity; this may cause him to be nonadherent to the rehabilitation protocol by engaging in activities not recommended by his sport medicine professional.
3. What strategies can the sport medicine professional incorporate into rehabilitation to keep Michael on track with his rehabilitation protocol?

References

Arnheim, D. D. and Prentice, W. E. (2000) *Principles of Athletic Training*, 10th edn. Boston, MA: McGraw-Hill.

Bassett, S. F. (2003) The assessment of patient adherence to physiotherapy rehabilitation. *New Zealand Journal of Physiotherapy*, 31(2), 60–66.

Bassett, S. F. and Prapavessis, H. (2007) Home–based physical therapy intervention with adherence-enhancing strategies versus clinic–based management for patients with ankle sprains. *Physical Therapy*, 87, 1132–43.

Belanger, A. Y. and Noel, G. (1990) Compliance to and effects of a home strengthening exercise program for adult dystrophic patients: A pilot study. *Physiotherapy Canada*, 43, 24–30.

Bohannon, R. W., Barreca, S. R., Shove, M. E., Lambert, C., Masters, L. M. and Sigouin, C. S. (2008) Documentation of daily sit-to-stands performed by community-dwelling adults. *Physiotherapy Theory and Practice*, 24, 437–42.

Boyce, D. and Brosky, J. A. (2008) Determining the minimal number of cyclic passive stretch repetitions recommended for an acute increase in an indirect measure of hamstring length. *Physiotherapy Theory and Practice*, 24, 113–20.

Brewer, B. W. (1998) Adherence to sport injury rehabilitation programs. *Journal of Applied Sport Psychology*, 10, 70–82.

Brewer, B. W. (2004) Psychological aspects of rehabilitation. In G. S. Kolt and M. B. Andersen (eds), *Psychology in the Physical and Manual Therapies*. Philadelphia, PA: Churchill Livingstone, pp. 39–53.

Brewer, B. W. (2007) Psychology of sport injury rehabilitation. In G. Tenenbaum and R. C. Eklund (eds), *Handbook of Sport Psychology*, 3rd edn. New York: Wiley, pp. 404–24.

Brewer, B. W., Andersen, M. B. and Van Raalte, J. L. (2002) Psychological aspects of sport injury rehabilitation: Toward a biopsychological approach. In D. I. Mostofsky and L. D. Zaichkowsky (eds), *Medical Aspects of Sport and Exercise*. Morgantown, WV: Fitness Information Technology, pp. 41–54.

Brewer, B. W., Avondoglio, J. B., Cornelius, A. E., Van Raalte, J. L., Brickner, J. C., Petitpas, A. J., Kolt G. S. and Hatten, S. J. (2002) Construct validity and interrater agreement of the sport injury rehabilitation adherence scale. *Journal of Sport Rehabilitation*, 11, 170–8.

Brewer, B. W., Cornelius, A. E., Van Raalte, J. L., Petitpas, A. J., Sklar, J. H., Pohlman, M. H., Krushell, R. J. and Ditmar, T. D. (2003) Protection motivation theory and adherence to sport injury rehabilitation revisited. *The Sport Psychologist*, 17, 95–103.

Brewer, B. W., Van Raalte, J. L., Cornelius, A. E., Petitpas, A. J., Sklar, J. H., Pohlman, M. H., Krushell, R. J. and Ditmar, T. D. (2000) Psychological factors, rehabilitation adherence, and rehabilitation outcome after anterior cruciate ligament reconstruction. *Rehabilitation Psychology*, 45(1), 20–37.

Byerly, P. N., Worrell, T., Gahimer, J. and Domholdt, E. (1994) Rehabilitation compliance in an athletic training environment. *Journal of Athletic Training*, 29, 352–5.

Crossman, J. and Roch, J. (1991) An observation instrument for use in sports medicine clinics. *Journal of the Canadian Athletic Therapists Association*, (April), 10–13.

Daly, J. M., Brewer, B. W., Van Raalte, J. L., Petitpas, A. J. and Sklar, J. H. (1995) Cognitive appraisal, emotional adjustment, and adherence to rehabilitation following knee surgery. *Journal of Sport Rehabilitation*, 4(1), 23–30.

DiFabio, R. P. (1995) Efficacy of comprehensive rehabilitation programs and back school for patients with low back pain: A meta-analysis. *Physical Therapy*, 75, 865–78.

Duda, J. L., Smart, A. E. and Tappe, M. K. (1989) Predictors of adherence in rehabilitation of athletic injuries: An application of personal investment theory. *Journal of Sport and Exercise Psychology*, 11(4), 367–81.

Evans, L. and Hardy, L. (2002a) Injury rehabilitation: A goal setting intervention study. *Research Quarterly for Exercise and Sport*, 73, 310–9.

Evans, L. and Hardy, L. (2002b) Injury rehabilitation: A qualitative follow-up study. *Research Quarterly for Exercise and Sport*, 73, 320–9.

Fisher, A. C., Domm, M. A. and Wuest, D. A. (1988) Adherence to sports-injury rehabilitation programs. *The Physician and Sportsmedicine*, 16(7), 47–52.

Fisher, A. C., Mullins, S. A. and Frye, P. A. (1993) Athletic trainers' attitudes and judgements of injured athletes' rehabilitation adherence. *Journal of Athletic Training*, 28(1), 43–7.

Flint, F. (1998) *Psychology of Sport Injury: A professional achievement self-study program course*. Champaign, IL: Human Kinetics.

Friedrich, M., Gittler, G., Halberstadt, Y., Cermak, T. and Heiller, I. (1998) Combined exercise and motivation program: Effect on the compliance and level of disability of patients with low back pain: A randomized controlled trial. *Archives of Physical Medicine and Rehabilitation*, 79, 475–87.

Garza, D. L. and Feltz, D. L. (1998) Effects of selected mental practice on performance, self–efficacy, and competition confidence of figure skaters. *The Sport Psychologist*, 12, 1–15.

Granquist, M. D., Gill, D. L. and Appaneal, R. N. (2010) Development of a measure of rehabilitation adherence for athletic training. *Journal of Sport Rehabilitation*, 19, 249–67.

Hammond, A. and Freeman, K. (2001) One-year outcomes of a randomized controlled trial of an educational–behavioural joint protection programme for people with rheumatoid arthritis. *Rheumatology*, 40, 1044–51.

Johnston, L. H. and Carroll, D. (2000) Coping, social support, and injury: Changes over time and the effects of level of sports involvement. *Journal of Sport Rehabilitation*, 9, 290–303.

Kolt, G. S., Brewer, B. W., Pizzari, T., Schoo, A. M. M. and Garrett, N. (2007) The sport injury rehabilitation adherence scale: A reliable scale for use in clinical physiotherapy. *Physiotherapy*, 93, 17–22.

Levitt, R., Deisinger, J. A., Wall, J. R., Ford, L. and Cassisi, J. E. (1995) EMG feedback-assisted postoperative rehabilitation of minor arthroscopic knee surgeries. *Journal of Sports Medicine and Physical Fitness*, 35, 218–23.

Lox, C. L., Martin Ginis, K. A. and Petruzzello, S. J. (eds) (2006) *The Psychology of Exercise: Integrating theory and practice*, 2nd edn. Scottsdale, AZ: Holcomb Hathaway Publishers.

Meichenbaum, D. and Turk, D. C. (1987) *Facilitating treatment adherence.* New York: Plenum.

Penpraze, P. and Mutrie, N. (1999) Effectiveness of goal setting in an injury rehabilitation programme for increasing patient understanding and compliance. *British Journal of Sports Medicine*, 33, 60.

Ryan, E. D., Herda, T. J., Costa, P. B., Defreitas, J. M., Beck, T. W., Stout, J. and Cramer, J. T. (2009) Determining the minimum number of passive stretches necessary to alter musculotendinous stiffness. *Journal of Sports Sciences*, 27, 957–61.

Scherzer, C. B., Brewer, B. W., Cornelius, A. E., Van Raalte, J. L., Petitpas, A. J., Sklar, J. H., Pohlman, M. H., Krushell, R. J., Ditmar, T. D. (2001) Psychological skills and adherence to rehabilitation after reconstruction of the anterior cruciate ligament. *Journal of Sport Rehabilitation*, 10, 165–72.

Taylor, A. H. and May, S. (1996) Threat and coping appraisal as determinants of compliance with sports injury rehabilitation: An application of protection motivation theory. *Journal of Sports Sciences*, 14, 471–82.

Udry, E. (1997) Coping and social support among injured athletes following surgery. *Journal of Sport and Exercise Psychology*, 19(1), 71–90.

Vitolins, M. Z., Rand, C. S., Rapp, S. R., Ribisl, P. M. and Sevick, M. A. (2000) Measuring adherence to behavioral and medical interventions. *Controlled Clinical Trials*, 21, 188S–194S.

Wiese-Bjornstal, D. M., Smith, A. M., Shaffer, S. M. and Morrey, M. A. (1998) An integrated model of response to sport injury: Psychological and sociological dynamics. *Journal of Applied Sport Psychology*, 10, 46–69.

PART 2

Psychological interventions in sport injury rehabilitation

5

GOAL SETTING IN SPORT INJURY REHABILITATION

Monna Arvinen-Barrow and Brian Hemmings

Introduction

Since the original work of Locke and Latham (1985), goal setting has become one of the most popular and widely used psychological interventions in sport and is often implemented by athletes with the aim of improving performance (Weinberg and Gould, 2011). Research has identified three different types of goals; namely outcome, performance and process goals (for example, Cox, 2007; Hardy, Jones and Gould, 1996). Outcome goals are usually focused on the outcome of an event such as winning or earning a medal and involve interpersonal comparison. In contrast, performance goals often involve intrapersonal assessment, as they are typically focused on achieving a particular level of performance in comparison to one's previous performances and not to that of other competitors. Process goals are focused on the actions and required tasks in which an individual must engage to achieve the desired performance outcome (for example, Cox, 2007; Hardy *et al.*, 1996; Weinberg and Gould, 2011). According to Cox (2007), when all outcome, performance and process goals are used in combination, athletes are more likely to experience higher levels of performance improvement and psychological development in comparison to when different goals (for example, outcome goals) are used in isolation.

Moreover, the mechanistic goal setting theory (Locke and Latham, 1990) proposes that a linear relationship exists between the above-mentioned goals and performance. According to the model, goals which are difficult yet realistic, specific and measurable lead to greater performance improvement than vague, easy and do-your-best goals, provided that the person who is trying to achieve the goals has accepted and taken ownership of the set goals. These theoretical principles have since been applied to the rehabilitation setting and research has shown that goal setting can also be of benefit to athletes when injured (see, for example, Beneka *et al.*, 2007). Since athletes are naturally goal driven (Heil, 1993b) and often accustomed to use goal setting on a frequent basis, using this technique in injury rehabilitation should not be difficult but may not always be apparent. The purpose of this chapter is therefore to discuss how goal setting might be applied within the sport injury rehabilitation context. More specifically, the chapter: (a) introduces the purpose of goal setting within the sport injury context; (b) discusses the ways in which injured athletes can benefit from using goal setting during rehabilitation; (c) introduces different types and levels of goals that might be beneficial during rehabilitation; and (d) outlines the basic principles of goal setting during rehabilitation.

Rehabilitation goal setting: the purpose

According to the integrated model of psychological response to the sport injury and rehabilitation process (Wiese-Bjornstal, Smith, Shaffer and Morrey, 1998), the use of goal setting during rehabilitation is a multifaceted construct. In short, the model proposes that injured athletes' use/disuse of psychological strategies (for example, goal setting, a behavioural response) can have an impact on an athlete's cognitive appraisal of the injury (for example, ability to adjust their goals or rate of perceived recovery), which can have an impact on their emotional responses to the injury (for example, feelings of frustration, anger and attitude). In a similar manner, the cyclical relationships between cognitions, emotions and behaviours also functions in reverse; the use of psychological strategies such as goal setting can also have a direct impact on an athlete's emotional response (for example, facilitate emotional coping), which, in turn, can then impact an athlete's cognitive appraisal of the injury (for example, facilitate cognitive coping), which, in turn, can affect behavioural responses (for example, facilitate behavioural coping). The model also proposes that these cognitive, emotional and behavioural responses are mediated by a range of personal (for example, motivation, existing psychological skills) and situational factors (for example, level of competition, sport medicine team influences; for more details on the model, see Chapter 3).

Given the above, it is apparent that rehabilitation goal setting can serve multiple purposes for the athlete. Since goal setting is a motivational tool that can effectively energise athletes to become more productive and effective (Locke and Latham, 1990), its main aim should be to identify clear objectives for the rehabilitation process to enable athletes to return back to full fitness both mentally and physically. At its best, a well-planned and structured goal setting programme facilitates full physical, psychological and performance recovery, and allows athletes the possibility to make substantial performance gains (Taylor and Taylor, 1997).

Rehabilitation goal setting: benefits to the athlete

Research on the goal setting process during sport injury rehabilitation has shown that it has multiple benefits to the athlete. For example, setting goals during rehabilitation has been found to have a positive effect on the athlete's physiological and psychological healing (Ievleva and Orlick, 1991; Taylor and Taylor, 1997).

According to Beneka *et al.* (2007), some of the benefits include pain management when obtaining normal range of motion, muscular strengthening and numerous sport-related skills. Moreover, it appears that goal setting has a positive effect on the overall injury recovery process, as it has also been found to enable faster recovery and return back to sport (DePalma and DePalma, 1989). More recently, goal setting has been found to impact injured athletes' attitude, successful appraisal/acceptance of the injury, overall confidence in the injury recovery, as well as adherence to the rehabilitation programme (Armatas, Chondrou, Yiannakos, Galazoulas and Velkopoulos, 2007).

Of all the benefits mentioned above, it has been suggested that the main reasons why goal setting appears to be useful for injured athletes during rehabilitation, is its positive effects on adherence (for example, Arvinen-Barrow, Penny, Hemmings and Corr, 2010; Niven, 2007). The relationship between rehabilitation adherence and goal setting has been well documented in the literature and research has found it to provide the athlete with a sense of achievement and accomplishment, which further increases adherence (Fisher, Mullins and Frye, 1993). Moreover, goal setting has also been found to facilitate athletes' levels of motivation, effort and persistence (Brewer, Jeffers, Petitpas and Van Raalte, 1994; Weiss and Troxel, 1986), which can also be seen as beneficial in enhancing adherence. Over time, the use of goal setting during injury rehabilitation is also thought to increase athletes' levels of self-efficacy and self-confidence, as well as decrease athletes feelings of 'unspiritedness' (for example, loss of motivation and apathy; Evans and Hardy, 2002a), which have been linked with increased adherence. Moreover, goal setting has been found to impact common rehabilitation objectives such as communication, rehabilitation outcome assessment, as well as increasing overall adherence (Playford, Dawson, Limbert, Smith and Ward, 2000). As research suggests that adherence is a key determinant of whether or not an athlete is able to cope successfully with their rehabilitation (Arvinen-Barrow, Hemmings, Weigand, Becker and Booth, 2007; Clement, Granquist and Arvinen-Barrow, 2013; Heaney, 2006; Lafferty, Kenyon and Wright, 2008), it would seem that the use of goal setting to increase adherence is positively indicated.

> *Goal setting is vital. . . and very useful, very effective . . . because it is certainly for something where they (the athletes) can measure it themselves and see how they are doing Monday, Tuesday, Wednesday, Thursday and then by Friday they are getting the results that they want, so I think that's, that's certainly vital.*
> *(A Chartered Physiotherapist, cited in Arvinen-Barrow et al., 2010)*

Types and levels of goals

As sport injury can impact an athlete physically (that is, restricts movement and use of the injured and/or the surrounding area), psychologically (that is, changes in mood), tangibly (that is, restricts the accomplishment of typical daily tasks) and even financially (that is, loss of income owing to inability to work), an awareness of different types of rehabilitation goals is imperative. According to Taylor and Taylor (1997), physical goals can enable a clear direction for the physical aspects of recovery, whilst psychological goals can assist with issues associated with motivation, self-confidence, focus, stress and anxiety. Equally, performance-related goals can benefit the athlete by identifying potential areas for improvement in different areas of performance (for example, technical and tactical development, specific physical conditioning, mental training, and return to form), which, during regular training, might not have received priority.

Although setting different types of goals can provide injured athletes with clear objectives (Flint, 1998), it is also necessary to think about how these goals can be accomplished. Given that the ultimate aim of any rehabilitation is to return back to full fitness and often this can be a long-term process, injured athletes also need daily encouragement to ensure adherence to the rehabilitation programme (Hamson-Utley and Vazques, 2008). Taylor and Taylor (1997) propose that, during sport injury rehabilitation, different levels of goals should also be considered (see Figure 5.1). Hence, they propose four levels of goals; namely recovery, stage, daily and lifestyle goals. Recovery goals are associated with the final level of recovery (long-term goals), stage goals consist of specific objectives for each of the different stages of rehabilitation (medium-term goals) and daily goals relate to daily objectives and targets for each rehabilitation session (short-term goals). Often, daily goals can be overlooked in a goal setting programme; however, they should be set to ensure that stage and recovery goals will be successfully attained. In addition, Taylor and Taylor (1997) recommend that goals related to the athlete's lifestyle should also be considered, as, often, existing lifestyle (that is, sleep, diet, alcohol and drug use, relationships, work and school commitments) can either assist or hinder rehabilitation adherence and, ultimately, have an adverse effect on recovery outcome. White and Black (2004) also recommend identifying and setting goals for employment, social and leisure activities and general household tasks as useful for injured athletes.

Using goal setting for rehabilitation: the process

Setting goals during injury rehabilitation should follow a systematic and organised sequence of events to increase its effectiveness. These events can be conceptualised in terms of four phases: 1) assess and identify athletes' personal and physical needs for successful rehabilitation and recovery; 2) identify and set appropriate physical, psychological and performance goals; 3) consider factors that may influence goal setting effectiveness; and 4) follow a step-by-step programme to integrate goal setting into injury rehabilitation. What follows is a more detailed description of the steps above to provide the reader with guidelines on how to improve the usefulness of goal setting in injury rehabilitation.

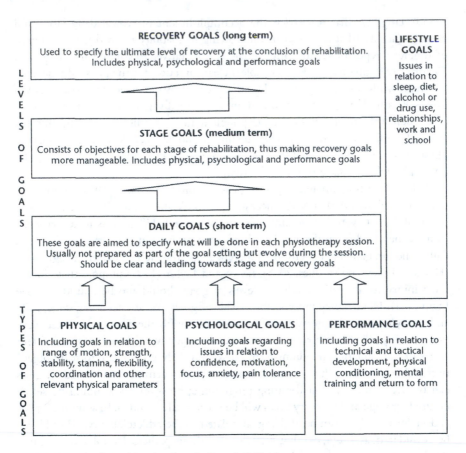

FIGURE 5.1 Types and levels of goals for rehabilitation

Source: adapted from the works of Taylor and Taylor, 1997 (Arvinen-Barrow, 2009)

Phase 1: Assess and identify athletes' personal and physical needs

One of the ways in which the assessment and identification of injured athletes' personal and physical needs can be facilitated is through the use of rehabilitation profiling (Taylor and Taylor, 1997). Founded in the principles of performance profiling (Butler, Smith and Irwin, 1993), rehabilitation profiling can help to gain an understanding of an athlete's perceptions of their current personal and physical factors influencing rehabilitation and recovery. Profiling enables injured athletes and sport medicine professionals to gain a visual display of a range of factors that are deemed to be important during the rehabilitation. Once these areas have been identified, they can then provide a foundation for subsequent goal setting for the sport medicine team (for more details, see Chapter 10).

Phase 2: Identifying and setting effective goals: key characteristics

Once the athlete's personal and physical needs have been identified, it is important to ensure that the subsequent goals are appropriate. A number of guidelines on effective goals have been proposed in the literature (for example, Cox, 2007; Gould, 1986; Heil, 1993b; Taylor and Taylor, 1997) and follow these general principles:

- understand the importance of setting the right type of goals;
- set goals that are specific and measurable;
- set challenging but realistic and attainable goals;
- focus on the degree of, rather than on the absolute, attainment of goals;
- set goals that are stated in a positive manner.

Understand the importance of setting the right type of goals

Flint (1998) argues that it is important to set both short- and long-term goals and, when possible, to link goals with aspects of the athlete's performance with which he/she is familiar (for example, designing goals to enhance important aspects of the athlete's sport). Flint also suggests that greater emphasis should be placed on process goals, since they are more likely to be within the athlete's own control and are directly linked with effort. More specifically, process goals should be linked with outcome goals and, as such, should be set for all levels of rehabilitation (short, intermediate and long term; Taylor and Taylor, 1997). Indeed, Evans Hardy, and Flemming (2000) found support for the use of long- and short-term goals, as well as process and performance goals.

Set goals that are specific and measurable

Locke and Latham (1990) proposed that vague and immeasurable goals are not as effective as specific and measurable goals. Without the ability to measure progress, the athlete may easily feel that rehabilitation is not progressing, thus leading to decreased levels of motivation and disengagement (a behavioural response), as well as negative changes in mood (an emotional response) and irrational thoughts associated with injury, recovery and self (a cognitive appraisal). Ensuring the goals are specific and measurable allows the injured athlete to evaluate progress and therefore sustain effort throughout the different phases of rehabilitation.

Set challenging but realistic and attainable goals

A number of researchers appear to be in an agreement that goals that are too easy or too difficult can lead to decreased levels of motivation and thus lead to the athlete 'giving up' before they even start (for example, Cox, 2007; Gould, 1986; Heil, 1993b; Taylor and Taylor, 1997). Ensuring that goals meet the athlete's needs is of particular importance during injury rehabilitation when their thoughts, emotions and behaviours may already be uncharacteristic to their typical responses, owing to the injury.

Focus on the degree of, rather than on the absolute attainment of goals

Despite the importance of setting goals with a clear timetable for completion, it is common for a rehabilitation process to progress faster or slower than originally predicted. According to Gilbourne and Taylor (1998), 'recovery is typified by an unpredictable mix of rapid progress and disappointing setbacks' (p. 135) and, as such, research tends to be in favour of adopting a flexible approach to goal setting during rehabilitation (Heil, 1993a). Therefore, emphasis should be on the degree of, rather than absolute, attainment of goals to ensure that they remain reachable and meaningful for the athlete (for example, making gradual percentage gains in range of motion). A qualitative study by Evans *et al.* (2000) found goal flexibility to be greatly beneficial during recovery setbacks and in dealing with unpredictable physical factors such as swelling, soreness and pain.

Set goals that are stated in a positive manner

Rehabilitation goals should also be set in a positive manner. Given that injured athletes may engage in negative self-talk during rehabilitation, using positive terminology in goal setting can also assist in challenging negative thoughts (for more details on self-talk in rehabilitation, see Chapter 8).

Phase 3: Identify and consider factors affecting goal setting effectiveness

In addition to ensuring that goals are set in an appropriate manner, there are a number of other factors that can have an impact on goal setting effectiveness that should be considered by those involved in the goal setting process.

Ensure that goal setting is fully integrated into rehabilitation

In order for goal setting to be successful, it is vital that injured athletes and sport medicine professionals both regard it as an integral part of rehabilitation. Goal setting as a psychological technique is easily paired with a behavioural outcome that can be directly linked to rehabilitation process or outcome (for example, setting appropriate rehabilitation goals will help speed up the recovery process and improve adherence). Motivating athletes and sport medicine professionals to use systematic goal setting should not, therefore, be difficult, provided that they are appropriately educated about the process and benefits of goal setting. Indeed, it appears that sport medicine professionals already display positive attitudes towards the use of goal setting (Arvinen-Barrow *et al.*, 2007; Arvinen-Barrow *et al.*, 2010; Hamson-Utley, Martin and Walters, 2008) and, owing to their usual close daily proximity to the injured athlete, they are in an ideal position to use systematic goal setting procedures effectively during rehabilitation.

Consider goal setting as an individualised mutual sharing and dynamic process

Flint (1998) believes that goal setting should include specific details on how goals are to be achieved and that this process should be educational. Sport medicine professionals involved in the process need to work together with the injured athlete to establish realistic goals for the rehabilitation programme (Kolt, 2004). Through a good understanding of the goal setting process and desired outcome, an athlete is more likely to comply with the rehabilitation programme. Involving the athlete will also facilitate greater levels of communication and increase understanding and awareness of the injury and rehabilitation process. Likewise, enhanced communication leads to better trust and rapport between athlete and support personnel. Moreover, goal setting during rehabilitation is also a process which evolves over time and is impacted by a number of personal (for example, injury factors and individual differences) and situational (for example, rehabilitation team influences) factors. Owing to this dynamic process, any goal setting during rehabilitation should be individualised and should attempt to incorporate all factors needed for a successful return to sport.

It appears that goal setting is often used during rehabilitation, although this may be in an unstructured way (for example, Arvinen-Barrow *et al.*, 2010). It appears that setting goals during rehabilitation is often sport medicine professional mandated, rather than a result of a mutual dialogue between the athlete and the sport medicine professionals (Arvinen-Barrow *et al.*, 2010). Moreover, sport coaches have reported the need to use goal setting during injury rehabilitation but their assistance has not been systematic in nature (Podlog and Dionigi, 2010). For goal setting to be effective, including the athlete, coach and relevant members of the rehabilitation team in the goal setting process is vital.

Understand the importance of goal acceptance/commitment

Gilbourne, Taylor, Downie, and Newton (1996) believed that, for goal setting to be successful, the athletes involved would have to accept the set goals, as, without goal commitment, goal setting would be ineffective. To increase commitment to rehabilitation goals, injured athletes need to feel that their opinions are valued and that their input is an integral part of the rehabilitation process as a whole (Wauda, Armenth-Brothers and Boyce, 1998). These feelings of shared ownership of a programme can facilitate higher levels of commitment and motivation, which, in turn, can increase rehabilitation adherence. Moreover, as goal setting is a process which should involve all those involved in the rehabilitation, it is equally important to ensure sport medicine professionals working with the athlete are also committed to the goals (Flint, 1998).

Monitor and evaluate set goals regularly

To maintain athlete and sport medicine professional commitment, to assess goal setting effectiveness and to ensure that goal setting is continually appropriate for the injured athlete in the different phases of rehabilitation, it is important to monitor, evaluate and adjust goals during the course of rehabilitation (Flint, 1998; Gould, 1986; Heil, 1993b). Through monitoring, evaluation and regular feedback, the injured athlete could be helped to understand and appreciate their progress and subsequently increase their feelings of personal achievement, motivation and attitude towards recovery. This can positively influence commitment, treatment compliance and adherence as well as overall recovery outcomes.

Prepare a written contract with the injured athlete

Commitment, adherence and motivation to work towards the set goals can be influenced by preparing a written contract to which both the athlete and the sport medicine professionals are bound. Moreover, when both parties are clear of the expectations placed upon them during rehabilitation, the recovery is likely to progress with fewer complications (Figure 5.2).

Be aware of variability in goal setting effectiveness

Despite the apparent benefits of goal setting during rehabilitation, it is important to note that it is not always effective. For example, Johnson (2000) investigated the effects of short-term psychological interventions on injured athletes' mood and found that when used in isolation, goal setting had no significant effects. However, when used in combination with other psychological interventions (for example, stress management strategies, self-talk, relaxation techniques or imagery), goal setting was found to have the potential to help elevate athletes' mood during rehabilitation.

Moreover, it is also important to note that not always do athletes and sport medicine professionals view the effectiveness of psychological interventions equally. For example, Francis, Andersen, and Maley (2000) found that sport medicine professionals regarded the use of short-term goals as an effective technique for treatment and believed that athletes who set goals during rehabilitation were more likely to cope better with their injuries. Conversely, the athletes in this study viewed goal setting as useful for coping with injuries but rated the importance of setting short-term goals considerably lower than the sport medicine professionals. Nevertheless, if the basic guidelines of systematic goal setting are followed, these differences in opinions about the effectiveness will be highlighted and, as a result, adjustments to the goal setting programme can be made to ensure that it meets the needs of all parties involved.

Injured athlete

I, _____ agree to diligently fulfil my responsibilities in the rehabilitation of my injury. These responsibilities include:

1. Taking full control of all aspects of my rehabilitation.
2. Precise adherence to the rehabilitation programme designed for me.
3. Attendance at all scheduled physiotherapy sessions.
4. Completion of all exercises outside the rehabilitation facility.
5. Full effort, focus and intensity with all aspects of my rehabilitation regimen.
6. Consistent pursuit of the goals I set in my rehabilitation goal setting programme.
7. Developing psychological areas that impact my recovery and return to sport (e.g. addressing re-injury anxieties).
8. Improving myself as an athlete during rehabilitation.
9. Seeking assistance from others when difficulties arise.

Rehabilitation professional

I, _____ agree to diligently fulfil my responsibilities as the rehabilitation professional in the rehabilitation of _____'s injury. These responsibilities include:

1. Designing an individualised rehabilitation programme for the injured athlete.
2. Educating the athlete about all relevant aspects of the rehabilitation process.
3. Helping to establish a series of goals that will progressively lead to full recovery and return to sport.
4. Creating a rehabilitation team with other relevant professionals.
5. Being sensitive and responsive to psychological and emotional needs.
6. Assisting the athlete in overcoming physical and psychological obstacles that may arise during rehabilitation.
7. Providing the athlete with the information and skills to facilitate physical, psychological and performance contributors to a successful return to sport.

Athlete	Date
Rehabilitation professional	Date

FIGURE 5.2   An example of a rehabilitation contract

Source: adapted from Taylor and Taylor, 1997

Phase 4: A step by step programme to integrate goal setting into injury rehabilitation

When setting goals for rehabilitation, the above principles can ensure goals are set appropriately for each individual in question. According to Taylor and Taylor (1997), the process for setting such goals should begin with a conversation between the rehabilitation professionals and the athlete in which critical physical aspects of rehabilitation are discussed and explained. This should then be followed by setting clear goals for each of the components of physical recovery: range of motion, strength, stability, stamina, flexibility, and any other relevant physical parameters. Psychological goals should then be discussed in a similar manner. One of the most effective ways to initiate psychological rehabilitation goals is through rehabilitation profiling (Taylor and Taylor, 1997). Secondly, strategies for achieving goals need to be agreed upon and learned by athletes. By doing so, the athlete is more likely to feel a sense of control (Boyle, 2003; Kolt, 2004), which has been found to have an effect on rehabilitation adherence. Thirdly, and perhaps most importantly, the set goals need to be revised and assessed on a regular basis in order for them to be effective (Gould, 1986). Butler (1997) indicates that this could be done through various methods, such as diaries, meetings, graphs, and rehabilitation contracts.

Process of goal setting during sport injury rehabilitation

1. Start with a conversation between the rehabilitation professionals and the athlete.
2. Set clear goals for each of the components of physical recovery: range of motion, strength, stability, stamina, flexibility and any other relevant physical parameters.
3. Discuss psychological goals in a similar manner by using a tool such as rehabilitation profiling (for more details, see Chapter 10).
4. Agree upon any strategies needed for achieving goals.
5. Remember to revise and assess your goals regularly.

(Taylor and Taylor, 1997)

Conclusion

The importance of setting goals during rehabilitation has been highlighted in the literature. Support for goal setting can be found in various studies investigating athletes representing a range of sports, and various competitive levels (for example, Bassett and Petrie, 1999; Brewer *et al.*, 1994; Evans and Hardy, 2002a, 2002b; Evans *et al.*, 2000; Francis *et al.*, 2000; Gilbourne *et al.*, 1996; Gould, Udry, Bridges and Beck, 1997; Ievleva and Orlick, 1991; Johnson, 2000). In summary, studies to date have indicated that using goal setting during sport injury rehabilitation is beneficial. For many injured athletes, the hardest thing is to try and pace their recovery appropriately and not to progress too fast (Samples [1987] cited in Wagman and Khelifa, 1996: 257). Through goal setting, appropriate pace of progression can be identified and monitored. Furthermore, goal setting often forms an integral part of an athlete's everyday training programmes. Thus, it makes sense to continue similar procedures during rehabilitation. For that reason, the integration of goal setting into the rehabilitation process is not only profitable but, with the right guidance and support, should also be easily transferable (Taylor and Taylor, 1997).

CASE STUDY

Marika is a 16-year-old, international-level synchronized skater who has recently suffered a grade III hamstring injury to her left leg. Her doctor and physiotherapist have told her that the recovery would take up to five weeks and she has been advised to use crutches to help her walk. Marika is ignoring her doctor's and physiotherapist's advice and is often found walking without using her crutches, particularly when at school. When asked about reasons as to why she is not using crutches, Marika replies: 'it's so much easier not to use the crutches, as that way I don't have to ask my friends to help me with minor things like carrying my lunch tray to the table...I mean, I am not crippled you know. And at school, the breaks are so short that by the time I call the lift, and it comes to my floor, and takes me downstairs, I would have walked the stairs up and down several times, and the break is nearly over. Yes, I do have an injury in my leg, but it's really not a big deal. I will be back skating in no time'. Six weeks later, Marika is still not fit to train. Her hamstring has not fully healed and it keeps swelling up after completing her rehabilitation exercises. Marika is getting frustrated and angry with the process and often takes this out on her mother and her 13-year-old brother Matti. This has obviously impacted on the overall mood in their home and resulted in Marika being really distant and uncooperative when at home. Marika is now refusing to do her home exercises and thinks watching daytime TV, eating crisps and chocolate is much more fun than doing the 'boring' rehabilitation exercises. The season is fast approaching and Marika does not think she is going to be ready to go back on the ice and does not believe that she will be selected to skate at the first competitions in three months time. 'I am just not good enough to skate; others know the programme much better than I do...so what is the point of even going to the rink if I can't compete?' These thoughts, along with spending time with her classmates who do not skate but spend their afternoons at the local shopping centre, has led to her thinking about quitting skating altogether. Marika's mother and father are obviously not happy with the situation, especially after they got a letter from her physiotherapist enquiring why Marika had missed her last three physiotherapy sessions, despite her parents paying them in advance.

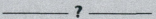

1. With reference to the integrated model of psychological response to sport injury and rehabilitation process (Wiese-Bjornstal *et al.*, 1998), what factors described in the case study may have affected Marika's cognitive appraisal of her hamstring injury?
2. What types of goals might be beneficial for Marika and why?
3. Following goal setting principles (Gould, 1996), set a variety of daily, stage, recovery and lifestyle goals to help Marika get back to skating and be ready to compete in three months.

References

Armatas, V., Chondrou, E., Yiannakos, A., Galazoulas, C. and Velkopoulos, C. (2007) Psychological aspects of rehabilitation following serious athletic injuries with special reference to goal setting: A review study. *Physical Training*, January. Retrieved from http://ejmas.com/pt/ptframe.htm

Arvinen-Barrow, M. (2009) *Psychological Rehabilitation from Sport Injury: Issues in training and development of chartered physiotherapists* (PhD thesis). University of Northampton. Available from http://nectar.northampton.ac.uk/2456/

Arvinen-Barrow, M., Hemmings, B., Weigand, D. A., Becker, C. A. and Booth, L. (2007) Views of chartered physiotherapists on the psychological content of their practice: A national follow-up survey in the United Kingdom. *Journal of Sport Rehabilitation*, 16, 111–21.

Arvinen-Barrow, M., Penny, G., Hemmings, B. and Corr, S. (2010) UK chartered physiotherapists' personal experiences in using psychological interventions with injured athletes: an interpretative phenomenological analysis. *Psychology of Sport and Exercise*, 11(1), 58–66.

Bassett, S. F. and Petrie, K. J. (1999) The effect of treatment goals on patient compliance with physiotherapy exercise programmes. *Physiotherapy*, 85(3), 130–7.

Beneka, A., Malliou, P., Bebetsos, E., Gioftsidou, A., Pafis, G. and Godolias, G. (2007) Appropriate counselling techniques for specific components of the rehabilitation plan: A review of the literature. *Physical Training*, August. Retrieved from http://ejmas.com/pt/ptframe.htm.

Boyle, S. (2003) Goal setting: The injured athlete. *Swim*, 20(1), 18–19.

Brewer, B. W., Jeffers, K. E., Petitpas, A. J. and Van Raalte, J. L. (1994) Perceptions of psychological interventions in the context of sport injury rehabilitation. *The Sport Psychologist*, 8, 176–88.

Butler, R. J. (1997) Psychological principles applied to sports injuries. In S. French (ed.), *Physiotherapy: A psychosocial approach*, 2nd edn. Oxford: Butterworth-Heinemann, pp. 155–68.

Butler, R. J., Smith, M. and Irwin, I. (1993) The performance profile in practice. *Journal of Applied Sport Psychology*, 5, 48–63.

Clement, D., Granquist, M. and Arvinen-Barrow, M. (2013) Psychosocial aspects of athletic injuries as perceived by athletic trainers. *Journal of Athletic Training*.

Cox, R. H. (2007) *Sport Psychology: Concepts and applications*, 6th edn. Boston, MA: McGraw–Hill.

DePalma, M. T. and DePalma, B. (1989) The use of instruction and the behavioural approach to facilitate injury recovery. *Athletic Training*, 24, 217–9.

Evans, L. and Hardy, L. (2002a) Injury rehabilitation: A goal setting intervention study. *Research Quarterly for Exercise and Sport*, 73, 310–9.

Evans, L. and Hardy, L. (2002b) Injury rehabilitation: A qualitative follow-up study. *Research Quarterly for Exercise and Sport*, 73, 320–9.

Evans, L., Hardy, L. and Flemming, S. (2000) Intervention strategies with injured athletes: An action research study. *The Sport Psychologist*, 14, 188–206.

Fisher, A. C., Mullins, S. A. and Frye, P. A. (1993) Athletic trainers' attitudes and judgements of injured athletes' rehabilitation adherence. *Journal of Athletic Training*, 28(1), 43–7.

Flint, F. A. (1998) Specialized psychological interventions In F. A. Flint (ed.), *Psychology of Sport Injury*. Leeds: Human Kinetics, pp. 29–50.

Francis, S. R., Andersen, M. B. and Maley, B. (2000) Physiotherapists' and male professional athletes' views on psychological skills for rehabilitation. *Journal of Science and Medicine in Sport*, 3(1), 17–29.

Gilbourne, D. and Taylor, A. H. (1998) From theory to practice: The integration of goal perspective theory and life development approaches within an injury specific goal setting program. *Journal of Applied Sport Psychology*, 10, 124–39.

Gilbourne, D., Taylor, A. H., Downie, G. and Newton, P. (1996) Goal setting during sports injury rehabilitation: A presentation of underlying theory, administration procedure, and an athlete case study. *Sports Exercise and Injury*, 2, 192–201.

Gould, D. (1986) Goal setting for peak performance. In J. Williams (ed.), *Applied Sport Psychology: Personal growth to peak performance*. Palo Alto, CA: Mayfield, pp. 133–48.

Gould, D., Udry, E., Bridges, D. and Beck, L. (1997) Coping with season-ending injuries. *The Sport Psychologist*, 11, 379–99.

Hamson–Utley, J. J., Martin, S. and Walters, J. (2008) Athletic trainers' and physical therapists' perceptions of the effectiveness of psychological skills within sport injury rehabilitation programs. *Journal of Athletic Training*, 43(3), 258–64.

Hamson–Utley, J. J. and Vazques, L. (2008) The comeback: Rehabilitating the psychological Injury. *Athletic Therapy Today*, 13(5), 35–8.

Hardy, L., Jones, G. and Gould, D. (1996) *Understanding Psychological Preparation for Sport: Theory and practice of elite performers*. Chichester: John Wiley & Sons.

Heaney, C. (2006) Physiotherapists' perceptions of sport psychology intervention in professional soccer. *International Journal of Sport and Exercise Psychology*, 4(1), 67–80.

Heil, J. (1993a) A comprehensive approach to injury management. In J. Heil (ed.), *Psychology of sport injury*. Champaign, IL: Human Kinetics, pp. 137–49.

Heil, J. (1993b) *Psychology of Sport Injury*. Champaign, IL: Human Kinetics.

Ievleva, L. and Orlick, T. (1991) Mental links to enhanced healing: An exploratory study. *The Sport Psychologist*, 5, 25–40.

Johnson, U. (2000) Short-term psychological intervention: A study of long-term-injured athletes. *Journal of Sport Rehabilitation*, 9, 207–18.

Kolt, G. S. (2004) Injury from sport, exercise, and physical activity. In G. S. Kolt and M. B. Andersen (eds), *Psychology in the Physical and Manual Therapies*. London: Churchill Livingstone, pp. 247–67.

Lafferty, M. E., Kenyon, R. and Wright, C. J. (2008) Club-based and non-club based physiotherapists' views on the psychological content of their practice when treating sports injuries. *Research in Sports Medicine*, 16, 295–306.

Locke, E. A. and Latham, G. P. (1985) The application of goal setting to sports. *Journal of Sport Psychology*, 7, 205–22.

Locke, E. A. and Latham, G. P. (1990) *A Theory of Goal Setting and Task Performance*. Englewood Cliffs, NJ: Prentice Hall.

Niven, A. (2007) Rehabilitation adherence in sport injury: Sport physiotherapists' perceptions. *Journal of Sport Rehabilitation*, 16, 93–110.

Playford, E., Dawson, L., Limbert, V., Smith, M. and Ward. (2000) Goal setting in rehabilitation: report of a workshop to explore professionals; perceptions of goal setting. *Clinical Rehabilitation*, 14, 491–6.

Podlog, L. and Dionigi, R. (2010) Coach strategies for addressing psychosocial challenges during the return to sport from injury. *Journal of Sports Sciences*, 28(11), 1197–208.

Taylor, J. and Taylor, S. (1997) *Psychological Approaches to Sports Injury Rehabilitation*. Gaithersburg, MD: Aspen.

Wagman, D. and Khelifa, M. (1996) Psychological issues in sport injury rehabilitation: Current knowledge and practice. *Journal of Athletic Training*, 31(3), 257–61.

Wauda, V., Armenth-Brothers, F. and Boyce, B. A. (1998) Goal setting: A key to injury rehabilitation. *Athletic Therapy & Training*, 3(1), 21–25.

Weinberg, R. S. and Gould, D. (2011) *Foundations of Sport and Exercise Psychology*, 5th edn.

Champaign, IL: Human Kinetics.

Weiss, M. R. and Troxel, R. K. (1986) Psychology of the injured athlete. *Athletic Training*, 21, 104–10.

White, C. A. and Black, E. K. (2004) Cognitive and behavioral interventions. In G. S. Kolt and M. B. Andersen (eds), *Psychology in the Physical and Manual Therapies*. London: Churchill Livingstone, pp. 93–109.

Wiese–Bjornstal, D. M., Smith, A. M., Shaffer, S. M. and Morrey, M. A. (1998) An integrated model of response to sport injury: Psychological and sociological dynamics. *Journal of Applied Sport Psychology*, 10, 46–69.

6

IMAGERY IN SPORT INJURY REHABILITATION

*Monna Arvinen-Barrow, Damien Clement and
Brian Hemmings*

Introduction

Many athletes, coaches and sport psychology professionals appreciate the usefulness
of mental imagery in enhancing sport performance (Hall, 2001). A wealth of
research evidence exists in support of imagery as being one of the most popular
performance-enhancement techniques in sport (for example, DeFrancesco and
Burke, 1997; Hall and Rodgers, 1989; Pain, Harwood and Anderson, 2011;
Weinberg and Gould, 2011). It appears that athletes of all levels frequently use
imagery (for example, Arvinen-Barrow, Weigand, Hemmings and Walley, 2008) and
that élite, high-level and successful athletes use significantly more imagery than
their novice, lower-level and less successful counterparts (for example, Arvinen-
Barrow et al., 2008; Callow and Hardy, 2001; Cumming and Hall, 2002a, 2002b).
It has also been found that the use of imagery goes beyond sport type classification
(for example, team vs. individual, open vs. closed, and fine vs. gross skill) as athletes
involved in a range of sports such as gymnastics, dance, figure and synchronised
skating, field hockey, rugby and martial arts appear to use imagery extensively (for
example, Arvinen-Barrow et al., 2008; Arvinen-Barrow, Weigand, Thomas,
Hemmings and Walley, 2007; Hall, Rodgers and Barr, 1990; Munroe, Hall, Simms
and Weinberg, 1998) and do so at different times of the season (for example,
Arvinen-Barrow et al., 2008; Cumming and Hall, 2002a; Munroe et al., 1998).
However, despite the documented use of imagery by athletes of different levels in
a variety of sports, using imagery during sport injury rehabilitation appears to be
largely underutilised (Walsh, 2005). This could be because of a lack of understanding of how imagery works in a rehabilitation setting (Arvinen-Barrow, Penny,
Hemmings and Corr, 2010; Brewer, Jeffers, Petitpas and Van Raalte, 1994; Walsh,
2005; Wiese, Weiss and Yukelson, 1991) or simply an indication of athletes' inability to transfer skills that they normally use for performance enhancement into

injury rehabilitation. This chapter discusses how imagery could be applied within sport injury rehabilitation context. More specifically, the chapter: (a) introduces existing definitions; (b) discusses the ways in which injured athletes can benefit from using imagery during rehabilitation; (c) presents the different types of imagery that might be beneficial during rehabilitation; (d) provides an overview of the existing research findings on each of the imagery types; (e) introduces the different functions of imagery; and (f) outlines the process of using imagery during rehabilitation.

Rehabilitation imagery: concept definitions

Morris, Spittle, and Watt defined imagery in the context of sport as:

> the creation or re-creation of an experience generated from memorial information, involving quasi-sensorial, quasi-perceptual, and quasi-affective characteristics, that is under the volitional control of the imager, and which may occur in the absence of the real stimulus antecedents normally associated with the actual experience.
>
> *(Morris, Spittle and Watt, 2005: 19)*

Similarly, Dent described imagery as:

> cognitively reproducing or visualizing an object, scene or sensation as though it were occurring in overt, physical reality. It evokes the physical characteristics of an absent object, event or activity that has been perceived in the past, or may take place in the future.
>
> *(Dent [1985] cited in Driediger, Hall and Callow, 2006: 262)*

Based on these definitions, imagery can be described in 'lay terms' as an activity which involves creating a clear mental picture of the sporting situations, which can mean the venue, the performance, the conditions, the people, the emotions and the feelings.

When applied to sport injury rehabilitation, imagery can be seen as an activity in which the athlete can create images of (but not limited to): the healing process, the injured body part fully healed and restored to normal levels of functioning, the rehabilitation setting, successfully completing rehabilitation exercises, dealing with pain and any emotions associated with the injury and recovery process.

Rehabilitation imagery: benefits to the athlete

As stated earlier, imagery has been found to be quite useful in the sporting context for maintaining and/or improving athletic performance. Furthermore, its applicability to injury rehabilitation is increasingly being documented in the literature, since imagery has been associated with facilitating the speed of physical recovery

(Beneka *et al.*, 2007; Ievleva and Orlick, 1991; Walsh, 2005), in addition to being deemed useful for athletes during the rehabilitation process. More specifically, imagery within in the context of injury rehabilitation has been found to:

- facilitate athletes' ability to better cope with their injuries (Gould, Udry, Bridges and Beck, 1997; Rotella, 1982) in addition to facilitating closure to their injury experience (Green, 1992; Green and Bonura, 2007);
- help athletes to manage the emotions, anxiety, worry and stressors typically associated with their injuries and the rehabilitation process (Hamson-Utley and Vazquez, 2008; Monsma, Mensch and Farroll, 2009);
- help injured athletes to deal with the pain associated with injuries (Hamson-Utley and Vazquez, 2008);
- assist athletes in eliminating counterproductive thoughts and aid in the development of a 'positive self' (Driediger, *et al.*, 2006);
- increase injured athletes' rehabilitation motivation and subsequently rehabilitation adherence and compliance (Hamson-Utley and Vazquez, 2008);
- prepare athletes for successful return back to pre-injury level of performance, both physically (that is, maintain sport-specific skills through the use of performance imagery) and psychologically (for example, assist in increasing levels of confidence, decreasing levels of re-injury anxiety; see, for example, Walsh, 2005).

Using imagery during rehabilitation

I think it's big. Especially just while doing the exercises and stuff because inevitably, well, especially after mine where I had the surgery and the muscles kind of went into atrophy... I had to reteach myself how to do things. And the only way I could do it, it's not like it's just going to happen and you can't rely on that. Or, if you do then it's just going to take a lot longer. So, it's kind of the same thing as with weight training, if you visualize it before, then you'll progress a lot faster and you'll start to see better results.

(An injured athlete, cited in Driediger et al.*, 2006: 267)*

Types of imagery

Thus far, a number of different types of imagery have been proposed as suitable and beneficial for rehabilitation. Drawing from the literature (Flint, 1998; Rotella, 1982, 1985; Rotella and Heyman, 1993; Taylor and Taylor, 1997), Walsh (2005) compiled the existing information and listed four main types of imagery beneficial to sport injury rehabilitation: (1) healing imagery (that is, visualising and feeling the injured body part healing), (2) pain management imagery (that is, assisting the athlete to cope with the pain associated with the injury), (3) rehabilitation process imagery (that is, assisting in dealing with challenges that athletes may encounter during the rehabilitation programme), and (4) performance imagery (that is, practising physical skills and imagining themselves performing successfully and injury free). The following section provides an introduction to each of these types of imagery.

Healing imagery

Healing imagery refers to images in which the athlete will see the injured body part healing (for example, imagining seeing ruptured muscle tissue getting better). According to Walsh (2005), healing imagery can be used to envision the internal processes and anatomical healing that take place during rehabilitation. Taylor and Taylor (1997) claim that, for effective healing imagery, an athlete must possess a full understanding of their injury and have the ability to recreate a realistic picture of the injured area. An awareness of the anatomical healing process and knowledge of the treatment modalities employed during rehabilitation is also essential. Furthermore, an athlete should know what the injured body part should look like once healed. Given the above, it can be assumed that engagement in successful healing imagery requires a fair amount of knowledge and training, which unsurprisingly requires some time and effort from the individual athlete and those involved.

Pain management imagery

Pain management imagery requires the injured athlete to create images of themselves free of pain. Of the six pain management techniques identified by Fernandez and Turk (1986; cited in Heil, 1993b: 163), pleasant imagining (visualising yourself in a comfortable and relaxed setting such as lying on a beach), pain acknowledgement (assigning the pain physical properties, such as colour, size, shape, sounds, feelings) and dramatised coping (pain seen as part of a challenge and reframing it as a motivational tool) are seen as most appropriate for sport injury rehabilitation (Walsh, 2005). All of the aforementioned types of pain management imagery can help injured athletes better cope with pain, reduce pain levels experienced and subsequently assist the athlete in dealing with a number of emotional and behavioural responses sometimes associated with injury.

Rehabilitation process imagery

Rehabilitation process imagery allows the injured athletes to create images of the many different aspects of rehabilitation process they could potentially experience such as completing exercises, adhering to the rehabilitation programme, overcoming setbacks and obstacles, maintaining a positive attitude and staying focused (Heil, 1993a; Ievleva and Orlick, 1991; Wiese et al., 1991). Moreover, this type of imagery can assist athletes in dealing with the challenges they may encounter during the course of the rehabilitation (Walsh, 2005). One of the ways in which rehabilitation process imagery is proposed to facilitate recovery is through self-efficacy. If an athlete believes and is able to visualise their ability to successfully complete an assigned rehabilitation task and/or exercise, he/she is more likely to be able to perform well and succeed. Green and Bonura (2007) argue that rehabilitation process imagery is central in a sport injury rehabilitation programme, as it can enhance athletes' motivation and subsequently have a positive effect on adherence.

Performance imagery

Performance imagery, through the mental rehearsal of sport-specific skills during rehabilitation, can help increase injured athletes' confidence in their ability to return to sport (Walsh, 2005). Furthermore, by imagining themselves back at play, injured athletes may report a decrease in the stress and anxiety that some may experience in the lead up to their return to play (Walsh, 2005). However, caution in the use of arousal-provoking images during rehabilitation is warranted, as they can result in heightened levels of somatic anxiety before returning back to sport (Monsma, *et al.*, 2009). Performance imagery can also help athletes to achieve major performance gains in areas which may not receive priority during regular training (Walsh, 2005). Moreover, as athletes often view injury as a hindering setback and as an obligatory and sometimes unnecessary time away from their sport (Taylor and Taylor, 1997), performance imagery can be useful in allowing athletes to recognise performance gains that are likely to increase their motivation and potentially improve the rehabilitation process (Richardson and Latuda, 1995).

Review of the literature of imagery type: an overview

This section provides a brief review of the literature on each of the imagery types presented above. While this review is not exhaustive, the primary goal of this section is to provide the reader with an overview of the research on imagery types and their effectiveness during rehabilitation.

To date, only a few studies have examined the possible benefits and effects of healing imagery in the rehabilitation context and on the recovery process (Cupal and Brewer, 2001; Handegard, Joyner, Burke and Reimann, 2006; Ievleva and Orlick, 1991; Loundagin and Fisher, 1993). The literature indicates that athletes who recovered faster have reported using significantly more healing imagery during the rehabilitation process than those who recovered more slowly, and that fast healing athletes also tended to take personal responsibility for their healing through the use of creative visualisation. When used in combination with relaxation and as an adjunct to physical rehabilitation, healing imagery has also been found to be beneficial in increasing knee strength, decreasing re-injury anxiety and lowering pain (Cupal and Brewer, 2001). Thus far, evidence (albeit very limited) exists in support of healing imagery facilitating physical healing. However, rather than focusing on the physical aspects of recovery, it has also been suggested that the effectiveness of healing imagery could also include psychological benefits.

However, to date, these have not been empirically tested (Walsh, 2005). More specifically, healing imagery may be beneficial to injured athletes in increasing self-confidence, motivation, rehabilitation adherence, anxiety control and ability to manage pain but, thus far, the beneficial effects of the above are merely anecdotal.

Similarly to healing imagery, little research has examined the effectiveness of pain management imagery in sport injury rehabilitation. Until now, existing studies have used different types of imagery as a means to alleviate pain but not specifically employed what is considered as pain management imagery. For example, Cupal and Brewer (2001) found reduction in pain as one of the main benefits of using a combination of relaxation and guided imagery when used in addition to physiotherapy. In contrast, a study by Christakou and Zervas (2007) investigated the effects of relaxation, together with pain management and rehabilitation process imagery and found no demonstrable effects of imagery on the reduction of pain. Despite the lack of empirical findings to support the use of pain management imagery for rehabilitation, leading authors in the field advocate the use of imagery (be it healing, pain management or other) as a means of alleviating pain during injury recovery and rehabilitation (Crossman, 2001; Taylor and Taylor, 1997; Walsh, 2005).

Research into rehabilitation process imagery also appears to be in its infancy. One of the few studies investigating the effects of rehabilitation process imagery was a longitudinal intervention study with a male rugby player with a severely dislocated shoulder injury (Vergeer, 2006). This study provided support for the use of rehabilitation process imagery, as the participant reported visualising himself making full(er) use of his shoulder. In addition, the participant also reported seeing himself performing at his pre-injury level of performance and imagining his injured arm copying the movements of his healthy arm during and after gym training. During the early stages of his rehabilitation, the participant often experienced involuntary replay images of the accident but, over the course of the rehabilitation, such images had virtually disappeared. He also explained how some of the images he was visualising were associated with physical sensations, such as visualising the movement of his 'bone ripping'. According to the participant, such images were also helping him to understand what had happened to his body, which, in turn, he felt was facilitating his recovery. Interestingly, over the course of the physiotherapy, these images diminished as the healing progressed. Despite being able to see his, head-of-the-humerus, bone ripping, the participant reported no use of healing imagery and, despite appropriate training, he was not interested in trying healing imagery as he felt that his injury was too complex and he was not physiologically knowledgeable enough to envisage the healing process appropriately.

Limited research measuring the effectiveness of performance imagery during rehabilitation exists (Monsma et al., 2009); however, the available research has typically been in support of its applicability for injured athletes. For example, Weiss and Troxel (1986) has highlighted the usefulness of visualising successful recovery (that is, performance imagery) during injury rehabilitation. Ievleva and Orlick (1991) found that athletes who engaged in performance (and healing) imagery recovered faster than those who reported less frequent or no use of imagery. Johnson (2000) found significant differences between the control group and the relaxation/guided imagery group (which consisted of mainly performance imagery with some elements of healing imagery). Some partial support for performance imagery was found by Christakou, Zervas and Lavalle (2007) as their results revealed significantly higher functional performance gains for muscular endurance for the imagery intervention group. In contrast, no significant differences for dynamic balance and functional stability were found. Imagery and relaxation techniques have also been found to be beneficial for the process of gaining a normal range of movement and during joint restoration process (Beneka *et al.*, 2007). Moreover, Monsma *et al.* (2009) found that imagining sport-specific images was more common amongst males than females and that it was more common before returning to sport than at the earlier stages of the rehabilitation.

Research findings have shown that there are four types of imagery which have been found to be useful in injury rehabilitation:

- healing
- pain management
- rehabilitation process
- performance

Sport injury rehabilitation: functions of imagery

Not only is it important to understand what (that is, the imagery type) is being imagined during rehabilitation, it is also useful to understand the different functions of imagery (that is, for what purpose is imagery used). Typically, the sport psychology literature has identified five types of imagery content as useful to athletes (Hall, Mack, Paivio and Hausenblas, 1998), namely cognitive specific imagery (imagining specific sport skills), cognitive general imagery (imagining executing entire plays/routines and sections of a performance), motivational specific (imagining winning a medal), motivational general arousal imagery (imagining controlling stress, anxiety and arousal) and motivational general mastery imagery (imagining feeling confident). However, very seldom have these imagery types been described in an injury rehabilitation setting (Monsma *et al.*, 2009) but rather the focus of rehabilitation imagery has been on the usefulness and effectiveness of healing, pain management, rehabilitation process and performance imagery during sport injury rehabilitation. The following section will introduce the research into the functions of imagery an individual athlete may use during injury rehabilitation.

Sordoni, Hall, and Forwell (2000) were the first to explore the functions of imagery use during rehabilitation. Their findings indicate that rehabilitation imagery serves both a cognitive and motivational function. In a subsequent study, Sordoni, Hall, and Forwell (2002) extended their earlier work by stating that injured athletes used imagery for cognitive, motivational and healing purposes. Milne, Hall, and Forwell (2005) supported the three-functional approach, as they found that athletes used significantly more imagery for motivational and cognitive purposes than for healing purposes. A link between imagery and self-efficacy was also found, as cognitive imagery was a significant predictor of task self-efficacy. Interestingly, in contrast, motivational imagery was not found to be a predictor for athletes coping self-efficacy, thus implying that motivational imagery is not as an important source of self-efficacy during injury rehabilitation as it is in a sport performance context. Driediger, *et al.* (2006) provided important information about how to build a foundation for imagery use during rehabilitation, as their findings revealed that athletes used imagery for motivational purposes, mainly in the form of reinforcing recovery goals (that is, imagining being fully recovered). Their findings also suggested that the actual imagery content also varied, as the athletes reported using different types of imagery; that is, healing, pain management and performance imagery (to learn and properly perform the rehabilitation exercises). In support, Evans, Hare and Mullen (2006) found that functions of imagery and imagery use varies depending on the rehabilitation stage of the athlete. It appears that during the early and mid-stages of rehabilitation, athletes appear to use healing, pain management and performance imagery, and that the performance imagery (cognitive specific imagery) is typically used for performance enhancement and not for rehabilitation. The use of cognitive specific imagery (that is, imagining successful execution of technical skills) was found to be as having a positive effect on the athletes' motivation, attitude and levels of self-confidence. During the latter stages, however, athletes appeared to use cognitive specific, cognitive general and motivational general mastery imagery and, overall, imagery was used mainly to maintain positive attitude and to increase self-confidence.

Drawing from the above, it is clear that imagery during rehabilitation can serve motivational, cognitive and healing functions. This can vary depending on the desired outcome and an athlete's personal and situational factors. Understanding the purpose of imagery use is important, as it can have an impact on the effectiveness of the chosen imagery type in achieving the desired outcome.

Using imagery for rehabilitation: the process

The incorporation of imagery into injury rehabilitation should follow a systematic and organised sequence of events to increase its effectiveness within the rehabilitation context. These events can be conceptualised in terms of two phases: 1) using a theoretical approach to determine the type of imagery to be used; and 2) following a step-by-step programme to integrate imagery into injury rehabilitation. It is advised that the above mentioned phases should be followed to increase the chances of injured athletes being able to maximise the benefits of imagery used during the course of injury rehabilitation. What follows is a description of the introductory steps and a brief discussion of guidelines to improve the usefulness of imagery in injury rehabilitation.

Using a theoretical approach to determine the appropriate type of imagery

Thus far, no clear theoretical framework for integrating imagery into rehabilitation exists. However, it is believed that, for the chosen imagery to meet athletes' needs and to ensure the effectiveness of the implemented imagery type, understanding how imagery works is essential. One of the most prominent frameworks for imagery use in sport is the applied model of imagery use in sport (AMIUS; Martin, Moritz and Hall, 1999). The model is centred around imagery type, which acts as a determinant to the possible cognitive, affective and behavioural outcomes of the imagery use. The model also proposes that the type of imagery used by athletes is dependent on the situation in which the imagery use occurs (that is, competition or training) and that athletes' imaging ability can act as a moderating factor affecting the imagery outcomes. It is believed that AMIUS could be also applied to injury rehabilitation imagery setting, namely to provide a framework for explaining the imagery phenomenon in injury rehabilitation and how to select appropriate imagery type during rehabilitation. Very similar to AMIUS, the aim of the adapted model is simply to describe how athletes use imagery during rehabilitation, rather than provide an explanation of the underlying processes of athletes' imagery use during rehabilitation (Figure 6.1).

When applying AMIUS to injury rehabilitation context, it is believed that the types of imagery (that is, what is imagined) would include healing imagery, pain management imagery, rehabilitation process imagery and performance imagery. These imagery types are directly linked with outcomes, which can include (but is not limited to): facilitating the process of physical healing, assisting the athlete in coping and dealing with pain, increasing rehabilitation motivation, adherence and compliance, maintaining sport-specific skills and strategies and assisting in physical and psychological preparation for returning back to sport. Moreover, the imagery types are also determined by the rehabilitation situation, which is closely influenced by the actual phases of rehabilitation and the stages of physical recovery (for more details, see Chapter 10). It is also believed that the effectiveness of the imagery type on the actual imagery outcome is mediated by imagery functions (that is, what purpose does the imagery serve?) as well as athletes' imagery ability (that is, what modalities are used for imagery?).

Sport medicine professionals who are interested in introducing imagery to their injured athletes need to consider the athletes' rehabilitation situation, imagery ability, imagery function and potential outcomes before selecting a specific type of imagery.

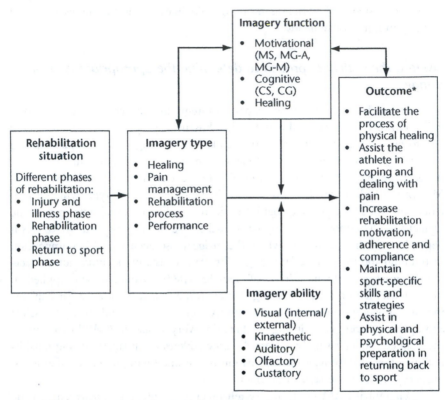

Note: * These are examples of potential outcomes and are by no means comprehensive; CG = cognitive general, CS = cognitive specific, MG-A = motivational general arousal, MG-M = motivational general mastery, MS = motivational specific

FIGURE 6.1 Application of the applied model of imagery use in sport into sport injury rehabilitation imagery

Source: adapted from Martin *et al.*, 1999

To determine which imagery type is most suited to the injured athlete, all of the above should be considered by those working with the injured athlete. It is proposed that those implementing imagery into rehabilitation should consider selecting the type of imagery based on the desired outcomes. This should also be affected by the rehabilitation situation, to ensure that the desired outcomes are realistic and purposeful for the phase of recovery. Moreover, consideration of the functions of imagery (that is, is the purpose of the imagery motivational, cognitive or healing?) as well as athletes' ability to imagine should be considered when designing and implementing imagery scripts during rehabilitation. Once the correct imagery type has been identified, those involved in the imagery process can move on to the second phase of the implementation by using a step-by-step programme to integrate imagery into the rehabilitation.

A step-by-step programme to integrate imagery into injury rehabilitation

Richardson and Latuda (1995) proposed a four-step programme showing how imagery could be integrated into injury rehabilitation. While this programme is very useful, the authors of this chapter have modified it to include an additional step, to ease any associated fears and concerns that sport medicine professionals may have about the incorporation of imagery into injury rehabilitation programs. The five steps are as follows:

1. Imagery should be introduced to the injured athlete with the intention of educating him/her about the practical application and potential benefits which could be derived from its incorporation into injury rehabilitation. Richardson and Latuda emphasised the importance of this step as they believe that 'imagery works the best when the athlete believes it will be beneficial to the healing process' (p. 11).

2. The athlete's imagery ability needs to be informally assessed. This can be achieved by asking the athlete some, if not all, of the following questions:
   a) what is your current use of imagery?
   b) describe your previous history with imagery.
   c) how often have you used imagery and in what context?
   d) how effective has your past use of imagery been?
   The information obtained from this assessment can then be used in the development of an imagery programme to be incorporated into the athletes' injury rehabilitation.

3. The athlete, depending on his/her history and experience with imagery, needs to be assisted in the development of basic imagery skills. Richardson and Latuda propose 15-minute training sessions twice daily. These sessions should focus on imagery vividness (the ability to create images that are vivid, clear and realistic in addition to incorporating all the senses; Taylor and Taylor, 1997) for a total of five minutes. Next, focus should be switched to image controllability (the ability to manipulate the image, making it do what they want it to; Taylor and Taylor, 1997) for five minutes as well. Finally, athletes should be exposed to self-perception of the image (for example, imagining their best ever performance, if relevant) also for five minutes.

4. Once the athlete is able to grasp a basic understanding of the skills introduced in the previous step, he/she needs to commit to practising the use of this skill until it becomes automatic. Practice should be encouraged in a variety of settings such as before, during and after rehabilitation-related activities and even in their personal time as well.

5. Once the athlete has put in the necessary time practising their use of imagery, it can be incorporated into their injury rehabilitation programme, making sure to keep the process as simple and concise as possible.

> The incorporation of imagery into injury rehabilitation should follow a systematic and organised sequence of steps to increase its effectiveness within this context.

Despite the aforementioned steps suggested above, it is also suggested that when integrating imagery in injury rehabilitation, sport medicine professionals should also be mindful of the following guidelines proposed by Taylor and Taylor (1997), which offer specific tips on how to maximise the rehabilitation imagery usefulness. These guidelines suggest that sport medicine professionals have the athletes:

- choose the imagery perspective (internal/external) which is most natural to him/her and then experiment with the other perspective;
- reproduce total performances. This means using all physical and psychological aspects of the injury rehabilitation experience;
- combine imagery with relaxation. The most important part of imagery should be to feel it physically and emotionally and such can only be achieved if your body is relaxed and your mind is calm;
- use imagery to facilitate physical and emotional wellbeing and feeling good.

Conclusion

Despite existing research being limited and on occasions lacking empirical rigour, rehabilitation imagery has the potential to be a practical psychological intervention technique to be used during sport injury rehabilitation. It has been argued that, during sport injury rehabilitation, imagery seems to serve four main purposes: to facilitate the actual healing process, to promote positive and relaxed outlook towards recovery, to create the required mind-set for optimum performance and to provide a closure to the injury experience (Green, 1992). This chapter has provided the reader with definitions of imagery in a sport injury rehabilitation context, highlighted the benefits of rehabilitation imagery to injured athletes and introduced the different types of imagery that might be beneficial during rehabilitation in addition to providing a brief overview of the research findings relative to each type of imagery. Moreover, the chapter introduced the different functions of imagery and outlined the process of integrating imagery into rehabilitation.

CASE STUDY

Stacey is a 25-year-old amateur golfer hoping to turn professional in the next 12–18 months. Her current handicap is 1, which according to her coach, is right on target with her long-term plans of turning professional. She has recently been diagnosed with a hernia in her groin and is now waiting for surgery scheduled for next week. She is experiencing a lot of pain and is worried that time away from practising before and after surgery will have an impact on her golf, particularly her short game routines. Until very recently, she has lacked confidence in her short game and the thought of not playing and practising makes Stacey feel very anxious. Her body feels tense and as she is constantly experiencing so much pain that her sleep pattern has become disturbed and the lack of sleep is making her irritable. 'I know I am very difficult to live with at the moment, but I just cannot help it. The pain at the moment is really bad and I think the pain relief is not helping. And what I think makes the matters worse, is the worry over losing my form. I just wish there was something I could do to make the situation a little more bearable at least'.

Her boyfriend is also a golfer, who has recently turned professional. Based on his own experiences, he thinks that Stacey might benefit from using some imagery to help her cope with the current situation. As Stacey has very little experience of using psychological skills, her boyfriend suggests that Stacey should talk to a sport psychologist he knows. Stacey reluctantly agrees, as she now thinks anything would be better than her current situation.

————— **?** —————

1. With reference to the integrated model of psychological response to sport injury and rehabilitation process (Wiese-Bjornstal *et al.*, 1998), outline key factors from Stacey's case study.
2. What types of imagery might be beneficial for Stacey and why?
3. Following the Taylor and Taylor (1997) suggestions, how could Stacey's imagery use during rehabilitation be maximised?

References

Arvinen-Barrow, M., Penny, G., Hemmings, B. and Corr, S. (2010) UK Chartered Physiotherapists' personal experiences in using psychological interventions with injured athletes: An interpretative phenomenological analysis. *Psychology of Sport and Exercise*, 11, 58–66.

Arvinen-Barrow, M., Weigand, D. A., Hemmings, B. and Walley, M. (2008) The use of imagery across competitive levels and time of season: A cross-sectional study amongst synchronized skaters in Finland. *European Journal of Sport Sciences*, 8(3), 135–42.

Arvinen-Barrow, M., Weigand, D. A., Thomas, S., Hemmings, B. and Walley, M. (2007) Elite/novice athlete's imagery use in open/closed sports. *Journal of Applied Sport Psychology*, 19, 93–104.

Beneka, A., Malliou, P., Bebetsos, E., Gioftsidou, A., Pafis, G. and Godolias, G. (2007) Appropriate counselling techniques for specific components of the rehabilitation plan: A review of the literature. *Physical Training*, August. Retrieved from http://ejmas.com/pt/ptframe.htm.

Brewer, B. W., Jeffers, K. E., Petitpas, A. J. and Van Raalte, J. L. (1994) Perceptions of psychological interventions in the context of sport injury rehabilitation. *The Sport Psychologist*, 8, 176–88.

Callow, N. and Hardy, L. (2001) Types of imagery associated with sport confidence in netball players of varying skills. *Journal of Applied Sport Psychology*, 13, 1–17.

Christakou, A. and Zervas, Y. (2007) The effectiveness of imagery on pain, edema, and range of motion in athletes with grade II ankle sprain. *Physical Therapy in Sport*, 8(3), 130–141.

Christakou, A., Zervas, Y. and Lavallee, D. (2007) The adjunctive role of imagery on the functional rehabilitation of a grade II ankle sprain. *Human Movement Science*, 26(1), 141–54.

Crossman, J. (2001) Managing thoughts, stress, and pain. In J. Crossman (ed.), *Coping with Sport Injuries: psychological strategies for rehabilitation*. New York: Oxford University Press, pp. 128–47.

Cumming, J. and Hall, C. (2002a) Athletes' use of imagery in the off–season. *The Sport Psychologist*, 16, 160–72.

Cumming, J. and Hall, C. (2002b) Deliberate imagery practice: The development of imagery skills in competitive athletes. *Journal of Sports Sciences*, 20, 137–45.

Cupal, D. D. and Brewer, B. W. (2001) Effects of relaxation and guided imagery on knee strength, re–injury anxiety, and pain following anterior cruciate ligament reconstruction. *Rehabilitation Psychology*, 46(1), 28–43.

DeFrancesco, C. and Burke, K. L. (1997) Performance enhancement strategies used in a professional tennis tournament. *International Journal of Sport Psychology*, 28, 185–95.

Driediger, M., Hall, C. and Callow, N. (2006) Imagery use by injured athletes: A qualitative analysis. *Journal of Sports Sciences*, 24(3), 261–71.

Evans, L., Hare, R. and Mullen, R. (2006) Imagery use during rehabilitation from injury. *Journal of Imagery Research in Sport and Physical Activity*, 1(1), Article 1. doi: 10.2202/1932-0191.1000.

Flint, F. A. (1998) Specialized psychological interventions In F. A. Flint (ed.), *Psychology of sport injury*. Leeds: Human Kinetics, pp. 29–50.

Gould, D., Udry, E., Bridges, D. and Beck, L. (1997) Coping with season-ending injuries. *The Sport Psychologist*, 11, 379–99.

Green, L. B. (1992) The use of imagery in the rehabilitation of injured athletes. *The Sport Psychologist*, 6, 416–28.

Green, L. B. and Bonura, K. B. (2007) The use of imagery in the rehabilitation of injured athletes. In D. Pargman (ed.), *Psychological bases of sport injuries*, 3rd edn. Morgantown, WV: Fitness Information Technology, pp. 131–47.

Hall, C. R. (2001) Imagery in sport and exercise. In R. Singer, H. Hausenblas and C. Janelle (eds), *Handbook of Sport Psychology*. New York: Wiley, pp. 529–49.

Hall, C. R., Mack, D. E., Paivio, A. and Hausenblas, H. A. (1998) Imagery use by athletes: Development of the sport imagery questionnaire. *International Journal of Sport Psychology*, 29, 73–89.

Hall, C. R. and Rodgers, W. M. (1989) Enhancing coaching effectiveness in figure skating through a mental skills training program. *The Sport Psychologist*, 3(2), 142–54.

Hall, C. R., Rodgers, W. M. and Barr, K. A. (1990) The use of imagery by athletes in selected sports. *The Sport Psychologist*, 4, 1–10.

Hamson-Utley, J. J. and L. Vazques (2008) The comeback: Rehabilitating the psychological injury. *Athletic Therapy Today*, 13(5), 35–8.

Handegard, L. A., Joyner, A. B., Burke, K. L. and Reimann, B. (2006) Relaxation and guided imagery in the sport rehabilitation context. *Journal of Excellence*, 11, 146–64.

Heil, J. (1993a) Mental training in injury management. In J. Heil (ed.), *Psychology of Sport Injury*. Champaign, IL: Human Kinetics, pp. 151–74.

Heil, J. (1993b) *Psychology of Sport Injury*. Champaign, IL: Human Kinetics.

Ievleva, L. and Orlick, T. (1991) Mental links to enhanced healing: An exploratory study. *The Sport Psychologist*, 5, 25–40.

Johnson, U. (2000) Short-term psychological intervention: A study of long-term-injured athletes. *Journal of Sport Rehabilitation*, 9, 207–18.

Loundagin, C. and Fisher, L. (1993) *The Relationship Between Mental Skills and Enhanced Athletic Injury Rehabilitation.* Paper presented at the Annual Meeting of the Association for the Advancement of Applied Sport Psychology and the Canadian Society for Psychomotor Learning and Sport Psychology, Montreal, Canada.

Martin, K. A., Moritz, S. E. and Hall, C. R. (1999) Imagery use in sport: A literature review and applied model. *The Sport Psychologist*, 13, 245–68.

Milne, M., Hall, C. and Forwell, L. (2005) Self-efficacy, imagery use, and adherence to rehabilitation by injured athletes. *Journal of Sport Rehabilitation*, 14, 150–67.

Monsma, E., Mensch, J. and Farroll, J. (2009) Keeping your head in the game: Sport-specific imagery and anxiety among injured athletes. *Journal of Athletic Training*, 44(4), 410–7.

Morris, T., Spittle, M. and Watt, A. P. (2005) *Imagery in Sport*. Champaign, IL: Human Kinetics.

Munroe, K., Hall, C., Simms, S. and Weinberg, R. (1998) The influence of type of sport and time of season on athlete's use of imagery. *The Sport Psychologist*, 12, 440–9.

Pain, M., Harwood, C. and Anderson, R. (2011) Pre-competition imagery and music: The impact on flow and performance in competitive soccer. *The Sport Psychologist*, 25, 212–33.

Richardson, P. A. and Latuda, L. M. (1995) Therapeutic imagery and athletic injuries. *Journal of Athletic Training*, 30(1), 10–12.

Rotella, R. J. (1982) Psychological care of the injured athlete. In D. N. Kulund (ed.), *The Injured Athlete*. Philadelphia, PA: Lippincott, pp. 213–24.

Rotella, R. J. (1985) The psychological care of the injured athlete. In L. K. Bunker, R. J. Rotella and A. S. Reilly (eds), *Sport Psychology: Psychological considerations in maximizing sport performance*. Ann Arbor, MI: McNaughton and Gunn, pp. 273–87.

Rotella, R. J. and Heyman, S. R. (1993) Stress, injury, and the psychological rehabilitation of athletes. In J. M. Williams (ed.), *Applied Sport Psychology: Personal growth to peak performance*, 2nd edn. Mountain View, CA: Mayfield, pp. 338–55.

Sordoni, C., Hall, C. and Forwell, L. (2000) The use of imagery by athletes during rehabilitation. *Journal of Applied Sport Psychology*, 3, 329–338.

Sordoni, C., Hall, C. and Forwell, L. (2002) The use of imagery in athletic injury rehabilitation and its relationship to self-efficacy. *Physiotherapy Canada*, Summer, pp. 177–85.

Taylor, J. and Taylor, S. (1997) *Psychological Approaches to Sports Injury Rehabilitation*. Gaithersburg, MD: Aspen.

Vergeer, I. (2006) Exploring mental representation of athletic injury: A longitudinal case study. *Psychology of Sport and Exercise*, 7, 99–114.

Walsh, M. (2005) Injury rehabilitation and imagery. In T. Morris, M. Spittle and A. P. Watt (eds), *Imagery in Sport*. Champaign: Human Kinetics, pp. 267–84.

Weinberg, R. S. and Gould, D. (2011) *Foundations of Sport and Exercise Psychology*, 5th edn. Champaign, IL: Human Kinetics.

Weiss, M. R. and Troxel, R. K. (1986) Psychology of the injured athlete. *Athletic Training*, 21, 104–10.

Wiese, D. M., Weiss, M. R. and Yukelson, D. P. (1991) Sport psychology in the training room: A survey of athletic trainers. *The Sport Psychologist*, 5, 15–24.

7

RELAXATION TECHNIQUES IN SPORT INJURY REHABILITATION

Natalie Walker and Caroline Heaney

Introduction

Several studies have explored the different stressors that athletes may have to cope with when participating in sport. The literature suggests that aspects of competition (for example, thinking about mistakes), interpersonal relationships (for example, expectations from coaches, team mates, or the media), financial concerns (for example, sponsorship), environmental conditions (such as the weather), and traumatic experiences (for example, enduring an injury), can all test an athlete's coping resources. The key to coping with these stressors is for the athlete is to learn to become self-aware of their responses to stressors and then adopt appropriate techniques (such as relaxation techniques) to facilitate coping. Thus far, a number of psychological interventions have been identified as being beneficial in helping athletes to deal with stressors, one of which is relaxation techniques. The use of such psychological interventions expands beyond the performance-enhancement context to also include sport injury rehabilitation (for example, Arvinen-Barrow, Hemmings, Weigand, Becker and Booth, 2007; Heaney, 2006). It has been documented that both athletes and sport medicine professionals use psychological interventions, including relaxation techniques, as part of rehabilitation programmes as well as during the process of returning to training and sporting competition following an injury. This chapter (a) introduces the purpose of relaxation techniques in sport injury rehabilitation; (b) outlines the types of relaxation techniques used in sport injury rehabilitation; (c) summarises the literature related to the use of relaxation techniques in sport injury rehabilitation; (d) discusses the ways in which relaxation techniques can be combined with other psychological interventions; and (e) provides practical advice to those working with injured athletes on how to maximise the use of relaxation techniques.

Relaxation techniques in rehabilitation: the purpose

Relaxation can be defined as a temporary deliberate withdrawal from everyday activity that aims to moderate the functions of the sympathetic nervous system which is usually activated under stress (Hill, 2001). When relaxed, individuals typically exhibit normal blood pressure and decreases in oxygen consumption, respiratory rate, heart rate and muscle tension (Benson and Klipper, 2000; Jacobs, 2001). When using relaxation techniques, the person should aim to learn how to voluntarily decrease the amount of tension in their muscles, calm their mind and decrease autonomic responses (heart rate and blood pressure).

It has been argued that relaxation techniques should form an integral part of the rehabilitation process (Flint, 1998) and a range of relaxation techniques have been identified as useful for injured athletes. For example, Flint (1998) suggests that progressive muscular relaxation (PMR), meditation, yoga, breath control techniques and autogenic training are useful. The literature proposes that these relaxation techniques are useful during injury rehabilitation for two primary reasons: firstly, to alleviate, control and assist athletes in coping with pain and, secondly, to reduce symptoms of stress and anxiety. Using relaxation techniques can also help to focus the athlete's attention, enhance confidence and aid healing, as well as to provide the athlete with a sense of control over rehabilitation.

Furthermore, many of the other psychological techniques that have been found to be useful during rehabilitation (such as imagery) actually rely on a foundation of relaxation to enhance effectiveness. Although presented separately in this book, the four principle techniques (goal setting, imagery, self-talk and relaxation) are readily integrated within a psychological skills training package when appropriate (for example, pairing relaxation with self-talk) and these methods are actually complementary. For example, relaxation training can be used to produce a relaxed state that is conducive to generating mental images for adopting healing imagery (see Chapter 6 for more details).

Useful relaxation techniques during sport injury rehabilitation

In sport, the term 'relaxation' or 'relaxation techniques' has been used to describe a range of methods through which an athlete can facilitate physical and psychological wellbeing. These methods are commonly split into two categories: physical (somatic) and mental (cognitive) relaxation (Flint, 1998). The primary aim of physical relaxation is to release physical tension in the body. In sport, the most commonly used physical relaxation techniques adopted are PMR (Jacobson, 1938), applied relaxation technique (ART; Ost, 1988), breath control techniques such as centering (see, for example, Harwood, 1998), diaphragmatic breathing (for example, McConnell, 2011), ratio breathing (for example, Dosil, 2006), and biofeedback (for example, Crews, 1993). In contrast, mental relaxation techniques focus more specifically on the mind rather than the body, with the belief that a relaxed mind will in turn relax the body. In sport, the main mental relaxation techniques employed are autogenic training (Schultz and Luthe, 1969) and transcendental meditation (Benson and Proctor, 1984). For the purpose of this chapter, the physical relaxation techniques of PMR and breath control (that is, centering, diaphragmatic and ratio breathing) are outlined, since these techniques have been shown to be particularly effective during sport injury rehabilitation (for a more detailed overview of the relaxation techniques, see Weinberg and Gould, 2011). In addition, the concept of mindfulness is also introduced to the reader as, within recent years, it has become increasingly popular amongst athletes. Mindfulness aims to increase awareness and attention, which is considered a predisposition for enhancing wellbeing.

Progressive muscular relaxation

PMR is the most commonly used and taught relaxation technique in sport (Flint, 1998). Based on the early work of Jacobson (1938), PMR aims to teach the individual what it feels like to relax, by contrasting the feeling of tension in specific muscle groups with the feeling of relaxation in those same muscle groups. Thus, the athlete becomes aware of when muscles are tense and, hence, when to relax them. PMR consists of learning to sequentially tense and then relax groups of muscles, while at the same time paying attention to both the feelings of tension and relaxation (Hill, 2001). Athletes are encouraged to observe early signals of stress and anxiety and to scan the muscles frequently for any tension experienced throughout the situation (for example, a rehabilitation session; Hill, 2001). The scanning required to perform PMR involves having the athlete note signs of muscular tension during the day and, by scanning the body at least twice a day, the athlete should be able to implement the relaxation response in a short time by using deep breathing (Crossman, 2001). When any tension is experienced, the athlete is instructed to tense these muscles, hold this tension for a count of seven and then release the tension, noticing the difference in sensation between tension and relaxation (Hill, 2001). In relaxing the musculature, it is believed that a calming effect occurs on the individual via the neuromuscular network (Payne, 2004).

When implementing PMR, after the initial deep breaths, subsequent breaths should be steady and shallow, with inhalations coming in through the nose and exhalations going out through the mouth (Crossman, 2001). The inhalation should lead smoothly into exhalation and not be forced or include a pause between the two (holding one's breath). The tension phase should last approximately seven to ten seconds and the relaxation phase should last approximately 25–30 seconds (Crossman, 2001). During the relaxation phase, the facilitator of the PMR (that is, the sport medicine professional) should have a lowered tone of voice compared with the tension phase (Crossman, 2001).

The first few sessions of PMR can take up to 30 minutes and it is recommended that athletes follow the PMR script for 16 muscle groups specifically when an athlete is learning PMR for the first time (Crossman, 2001). With practice, less time is necessary and the aim is for the athlete to be able to develop the ability to relax quickly (for an example PMR script see Weinberg and Gould, 2011). PMR is also commercially available in various audio formats (for example, CD, MP3, mobile applications) which could be used in sport settings and these may be facilitative (Taylor and Taylor, 1997). However, caution must be taken when selecting these sources to ensure that they are fit for purpose and should consider the perceptions of the athlete of the source.

Ost (1988) developed an applied variant of the PMR technique with the aim of teaching an athlete to relax within 20 minutes to 30 seconds. The first phase of training involves a 15-minute PMR routine practised twice a day. The individual then moves on to a 'release-only' phase (that is, muscle relaxation without deliberate prior muscle tension) that takes five to seven minutes to complete. This time is then reduced to two to three minutes, using the instructional cue 'relax'. This time is then further reduced until only a few seconds are required and then the technique is practiced for specific situations (between rehabilitation exercises). Eventually, the athlete is able to initiate a fast relaxation response as and when required, which is clearly of benefit to the rehabilitation process and beyond.

Learning to use PMR takes time and practice. PMR involves learning how to relax the whole body, and can take up to 30 minutes to complete.

Breath control techniques

Correct breathing is fundamental to achieving a relaxed state. A link exists between breathing and the system controlling our physiological arousal system. Stimulation of the sympathetic nervous system (when anxious) leads to breaths that are short, shallow and irregular and stimulation of the parasympathetic nervous system (calm and confident) is associated with smooth, deep and rhythmic breaths (Keable, 1989). This connection has created a perception that slow breathing has stress-relieving properties and, as such, one of the easiest yet most effective ways to control stress, anxiety and muscle tension (Weinberg and Gould, 2011).

Breath control techniques typically begin with exploring thoracic and abdominal movements when breathing leading up to a variety of different methods of breathing (for example, slow rhythmic breathing, deep breathing, diaphragmatic (abdominal) breathing, breathing meditation and ratio breathing; Payne, 2004). For the purposes of this chapter, centering, diaphragmatic and ratio breathing are described, as they are particularly effective during sport injury rehabilitation.

Centering

Centering is about focusing ones attention on the task at hand. There is a variety of different ways to centre but the most common appears to be changing the focus of attention from the athlete's head to their centre of gravity, hence giving a feeling of stability and balance. This feeling of stability, balance and control is the prompt to relax (Harwood, 1998). One key feature of centering is that, over time, with practice, it provides a method of relaxing quickly. A deep breath is all that is needed for the athlete to remove the feelings of anxiety (for example, on a new, more challenging rehabilitation exercise producing re-injury anxiety) and they can then refocus their attention on what needs to be done and how they are going to do it rather than on the possible negative consequences.

Sample centering exercise

- Stand with your feet shoulder-width apart and bend the knees slightly.
- Relax the neck, arms and shoulder muscles.
- Direct your thoughts inwards to check and alter your muscle tension and breathing, by focusing on the abdominal muscles and how they expand as you breath in. Try to feel the heaviness in your muscles.
- Take a slow, deep breath (from the diaphragm), trying to limit the movement of the chest cavity.
- Concentrate on your breathing and the heaviness of your muscles, clearing the mind of all irrelevant thoughts, and say 'relax'.
- Now focus your attention on the rehabilitation activity and what you need to do to perform it.

(Adapted from Harwood, 1998)

Diaphragmatic breathing

Diaphragmatic breathing emphasises the downward expansion of the chest cavity that causes the abdomen to swell. The first step in diaphragmatic breathing (and in all other breath control techniques) is to guide the athlete to become aware of their regular breathing patterns. Such can be achieved by completing the diaphragmatic breathing exercise steps shown here.

When engaging in diaphragmatic breathing exercises, if the athlete's chest rises more than their abdomen they should be shown how they might breathe differently and should have the benefits of this change explained to them. The aim of diaphragmatic breathing is for the athlete to try to feel their ribs expanding and moving as air is inhaled and then the ribs recoiling as they exhale. The athlete should be aware of how the lungs and diaphragm work. For example, athletes should know that the diaphragm forms the roof of the abdomen and, at rest, it is domed in shape. When it is contracted, it flattens, making more room in the chest for air to be inhaled. When the diaphragm is relaxed, it returns back to its dome shape, helping to force the air out. The movement of the diaphragm affects the position of the internal organs and, hence, when contracted it pushes down on these organs and causes the abdomen to swell a little. Injured athletes might find diaphragmatic breathing useful just prior to a rehabilitation exercise, to relax them in preparation for the exercise and to focus their attention on the task at hand. Diaphragmatic breathing can also be encouraged during the rehabilitation activities itself (the speed, agility, quickness work in the functional phase of rehabilitation) to improve the intensity and effort of the work.

Diaphragmatic breathing exercise

- Lie on your back (no postural effort needed from breathing muscles and organs shift, so diaphragm has something to work against and it is easier to learn in this position) and take small breaths in via the nose and exhale out of the mouth letting air just fall out of the lungs (do not force it).

- Gradually increase the size of your breaths until slow and deep (no holding of breath).

- You should be taking a maximum 12 breaths (inhale/exhale) per minute.

- Place the palm of your hands on the bottom of your ribs with the fingertips touching.

- On exhaling, relax the abdomen, shoulders and chest.

- Take in a big breath via the nose and notice what happens to the abdomen and ribs (for many, the chest will rise more than the abdomen).

Note: It is also possible to use paper or plastic cups instead of using the hands, for a more visual impact of current breathing patterns. Similarly, it is possible to replicate this exercise standing. For example, in front of mirror without upper body clothing; place your hands flat against your stomach (palms on bottom of ribs with finger tips touching).

(Adapted from McConnell; 2011)

Ratio breathing

Ratio breathing is a deep-breathing technique, with a focus on the number of inhalations compared with exhalations (for example, a ratio of four inhalations to seven exhalations). The individual counts the ratio of breaths and this is particularly useful for distracting from negative automatic thoughts. This can be easily explained to an athlete by using visual images. So, for example, asking the athlete to think of an open palm and to think of the counting of their breaths as the gaps between their fingers acting as a distraction to counterproductive thoughts. To demonstrate the opposite scenario, ask them to view the process by thinking of a fist and explaining that, when they are anxious, their negative thoughts enter their brain in quick succession and there is no intervention to slow them or stop these counterproductive thoughts.

It is also useful for the athlete practising ratio breathing to understand the arousal mechanism that ratio breathing is aimed to affect. The athlete engaged in ratio breathing should understand that an individual's levels of arousal are controlled by our autonomic nervous system, which is not under our conscious control. As such, what happens in our bodies is not typically what an individual might want to happen (for example, increased heart rate, increased breathing rate). When arousal levels are heightened, an individual needs to activate the parasympathetic nervous system, which is associated with a relaxed state. This can be achieved through taking slow, controlled longer 'out' breaths (hence, the longer exhale ratio compared with inhalation). One analogy that might be useful in explaining the above is the 'throttle and brake in a car' example.

> Being anxious is like putting your foot down on the throttle and letting the car get out of control. What you need to do is to put your foot on the brake and slow it down. Using ratio breathing is like pushing on that brake pedal and gaining control of the situation again.

Unfortunately, many individuals do not know how to breathe correctly. Some sport participants (for example, golf, pistol shooting, archery) are accustomed to engaging in such techniques, as correct breathing is often an integral part of successful skill execution. The sport medicine professional should pay attention to the individual's experience of such techniques when discussing breath control interventions during injury rehabilitation.

Mindfulness

In recent years, mindfulness has become increasingly popular amongst athletes. Cottraux (2007; cited in Bernier, Thienot, Codron and Fournier, 2009: 320) has defined mindfulness as 'a mental state resulting from voluntarily focusing one's attention on one's present experience in its sensorial, mental, cognitive and emotional aspects, in a non-judgmental way'. Mindfulness has its roots in Eastern meditational practice and, until recently, has been a relatively unfamiliar concept in Western culture. As previously stated, it is said to be a distinct form of awareness and attention, which could be considered a predisposition for enhancing wellbeing (Brown and Ryan, 2003). It uses breathing methods, guided imagery and other practices to relax the body and mind and help to reduce stress. Meditation exercises encourage individuals to engage in non-judging awareness of their internal experience occurring at each moment, such as bodily sensations, cognitions and emotions, and to environmental stimuli, such as sights and sounds (Baer, 2003; Kabat-Zinn, 1994). Researchers who have introduced mindfulness practice in mental health treatment programmes have taught these skills independently of the religious and cultural traditions (Linehan [1993] cited in Moore, 2009: 292; 295) and have developed several clinical interventions based on mindfulness training for anxiety, chronic pain, depression and post traumatic stress disorder (Garcia, Villa, Cepeda, Cueto and Montes, 2004; Ma and Teasdale, 2000).

Recent studies in sport psychology have also established a relationship between mindfulness and peak performance (Gardner and Moore, 2004, 2006; Kee and Wang, 2008). The ability to remain focused on the present has been found to be particularly important for performance outcomes. In the context of injury rehabilitation, mindfulness can be seen as beneficial to help injured athletes in achieving a relaxed state of mind and body and to become more aware of their injury situation. It may be useful in drawing an athlete's focus to the private events that they are experiencing throughout their rehabilitation, as well as encouraging such events to come and go without trying to control the experiences (Mahoney and Hanrahan, 2011). Mindful attention may also be useful to draw their focus to rehabilitation exercises to ensure correct execution of movements and to gain maximum benefits from physical interventions (Mahoney and Hanrahan, 2011).

Thus far, one study has explored the experiences of injured athletes during their rehabilitation from anterior cruciate ligament injuries and examined the usefulness of a mindfulness intervention, namely an adapted acceptance–commitment therapy (ACT) intervention in addressing individuals' adherence to rehabilitation protocols and their general psychological wellbeing (Mahoney and Hanrahan, 2011). Results highlighted that mindfulness was useful in accepting emotions such as frustration, boredom and anxiety. The authors also proposed that their findings tentatively suggest that an ACT-based educational programme may assist in the development of committed rehabilitation behaviours and the wellbeing of injured athletes.

> It has made me more aware of what is going on ... it's like you can pull away and be like, 'okay, it's just a thought, that's all it is' and then look at it a different way.
> (An injured athlete, cited in Mahoney and Hanrahan, 2011: 266)

However, as the research on the usefulness of mindfulness in sport injury rehabilitation context is in its infancy and as mindfulness is not a technique as such but a mental state which requires practice, encouraging athletes to use mindfulness to help in coping with injury rehabilitation should be reserved for those who have prior experience of using it.

A brief review of literature on relaxation techniques in sport injury rehabilitation

As stated above, a number of rehabilitation techniques have been found to be beneficial during injury rehabilitation. Based on the findings, these techniques can be typically grouped into three main areas: (1) dealing with pain, (2) alleviating stress and anxiety, and (3) increasing an injured athlete's focus, self-confidence and personal control during rehabilitation. This section provides a brief review of the literature in these areas and offers suggestions on how to use relaxation techniques during sport injury rehabilitation.

The use of relaxation for dealing with pain

Several studies exploring the effects of pain management techniques in a wide range of settings have indicated that an individual's overall pain tolerance can be improved and perceptions of pain reduced via the use of relaxation training (Caroll and Seers, 1998; Jessup and Gallegos, 1994; Linton, 1994; Owens and Ehrenreich, 1991), which may reduce the need for pain relieving medication (Payne, 2004). Pain inhibits breathing, reduces blood flow and can cause muscle spasms and tension. This can actually serve to increase pain in the long term (Cousin and Philips, 1985). Relaxation is hypothesised to affect pain via: 1) reducing the demand for oxygen in the tissue and lowering levels of chemicals (such as lactic acid) that can trigger pain, 2) releasing tension in the skeletal muscle that can exacerbate pain, and 3) the release of endorphins which interact with the opiate receptors in the brain to reduce perceptions of pain (McCaffery and Pasero, 1999). Another mechanism by which relaxation might reduce pain is via acting as an internal distraction. For example, if an injured athlete is engaging in ratio breathing, they might focus less on the pain itself and more on the breathing technique. For an individual experiencing pain during the night, relaxation techniques might also be particularly useful in facilitating sleep. Muscle relaxation can reduce the pain experienced and produces both a physiologically and psychologically induced relaxed state, making sleep more likely for the individual.

Injured athletes are likely to experience anxieties and fears associated with pain, which could potentially inhibit rehabilitation. Sport medicine professionals can therefore use relaxation techniques to reduce these anxieties (Christakou and Lavallee, 2009). Improvements have also been reported for pain, oedema and range of motion after a relaxation, pain management and imagery intervention (Christakou and Zervas, 2007). More recently, Naoi and Ostrow (2008) explored the effects of breathing techniques and autogenic training on injured athletes' mood and pain during rehabilitation. Improvements in mood and/or levels of pain were reported during the treatment period in comparison with the baseline control period. There was also some further benefit reported by the athletes with claims of improved physical and psychological recovery.

> I find that integrating relaxation techniques into my treatment sessions really helps get the most out of a session. I get my athletes to use a breathing technique before I start a treatment that might be a little painful and I find that it allows me to go a little deeper or a little longer. I don't know if it's the breathing itself or just giving the athlete something to focus on, but it definitely works!
>
> *(Megan, sport medicine professional)*

The use of relaxation to alleviate stress and anxiety

In addition to managing pain, relaxation techniques have also been found useful for controlling stress and anxiety symptoms (Taylor and Taylor, 1997). Relaxation techniques represent one of the most commonly used approaches in anxiety management worldwide, both as a stand-alone treatment or included in a more multimodal treatment (Manzoni, Pagnini, Castelnuovo and Molinari, 2008). Despite ones' best efforts, it is likely that at some time during rehabilitation the athlete will experience some form of stress and anxiety associated with their injury experience (Taylor and Taylor, 1997). Typical anxieties with which an athlete might have to cope include those related to the pain they are experiencing, lengthy rehabilitation anxieties, the loss of their starting place and change in daily routines, performance outcome anxieties (team doing well or poorly whilst injured), pre- and/or postoperative stress, anxieties related to fitness demands and returning to peak performance and also anxieties related to re-injury during rehabilitation or return to training and competition. These stressors can interfere with recovery because the healing mechanisms of body cannot work properly and to maximise the effects of treatment an athlete should be relaxed (Payne, 2004). When someone is anxious, one symptom experienced is excessive muscle tension and this might prevent the sport medicine professional from treating the injured area effectively. In addition, the injured athlete might also brace their muscles during a rehabilitation exercise in an attempt to protect their injured limb (Heil, 1993). This muscle tension can have a pain-enhancing effect in addition to reducing the flow of blood, reducing range of movement and increasing the risk of re-injury (Heil, 1993). As a consequence, the athlete might also experience lowered confidence, as they have little perceived control over their own body, and these symptoms might also interfere with their attention and concentration during rehabilitation exercises and, hence, increasing the risk of re-injury further.

As detailed earlier, an athlete might experience anxieties related to their injury rehabilitation and return to training and competition following injury. The use of relaxation techniques during these circumstances is vital. Relaxation training, such as PMR, is useful, as it increases the athletes' awareness of their muscle physiology. For example, an athlete might inappropriately believe that they are relaxed when in fact they are very tense but with the use of relaxation training they are able to gain greater sensitivity to their body and are hence enabled to become more in control. The use of breathing techniques and PMR are reported to be the most beneficial techniques for coping with stress and anxiety associated with injury (Wagman and Khelifa, 1996).

Deep breathing has been proposed as one of the simplest and most effective ways to reduce anxiety during rehabilitation by relaxing the muscles and subsequently relieving muscle tension (Taylor and Taylor, 1997, 1998). Cupal and Brewer (2001) investigated the effects of breath-assisted relaxation and guided imagery on knee strength, re-injury anxiety and perceived pain for athletes with anterior cruciate ligament injuries. They found that increased knee strength, decreases in re-injury anxiety and lowered perceptions of pain were evident in the treatment condition compared with the placebo and control conditions. Relaxation paired with imagery exercises can also be used to enable injured athletes to see themselves performing without anxieties (Flint, 2007; Green and Bonura, 2007; Walker, 2006; Williams and Andersen, 2007). The reduction in the negative effects of anxiety (reducing tension, decreasing blood pressure, lowering the heart rate, slowing breathing and increasing blood flow) can also have the potential to promote recovery.

The use of relaxation to enhance healing, increase focus, self-confidence, and personal control

Relaxation techniques can be useful in promoting blood flow to the injured limb, thus promoting healing and reducing the likelihood of re-injury (Heil, 1993; Taylor and Taylor, 1997). Furthermore, Beneka *et al.* (2007) suggest that relaxation techniques are also useful when the aim of the rehabilitation exercise is to obtain normal range of movement or restore joint stability and, hence, these techniques are very useful for promoting physical recovery. As a result of the direct impact of relaxation techniques on injury recovery, it is likely that an athletes' ability to focus, their feelings of self-confidence and personal control will be enhanced. The ability to adopt relaxation techniques can help the athlete to have a greater focus on the task at hand during rehabilitation by redirecting their attention away from discomfort, pain or anxiety and, ultimately, reducing the risk of re-injury. By controlling pain, discomfort and anxiety, it will provide the athlete with a sense of achievement, which in turn can enhance confidence. Moreover, all of the above will give the athlete a sense of personal control, which is often desired by injured athletes (Walker, 2006). Yukelson and Murphy (1993) stated that being an active participant in and having some responsibility for rehabilitation encourages positive involvement in the process.

An additional advantage of using relaxation techniques during rehabilitation is that when returning to their sport following recovery the athlete can also use these techniques in training and competition. These techniques can also help athletes in coping with other stressful situations and thus prevent any future injury/re-injury (for more details on stress-injury relationship, see Chapter 2).

Relaxation techniques can aid rehabilitation from injury by:

- helping the injured athlete deal with pain
- alleviating stress and anxiety, and
- increasing the injured athlete's focus, self-confidence and personal control during rehabilitation.

Pairing relaxation techniques with other psychological techniques

As previously stated, relaxation techniques are often used with other psychological techniques. For example, an injured athlete might be encouraged to select a word that is synonymous with relaxation (for example, relax, calm, healing, curing, peace, harmony) and to recite this cue word on exhaling (that is, pair relaxation with self-talk/cue words). The idea is that an association builds between the state of relaxation and the cue word and, over time, the cue word on its own can induce a relaxed state. The stronger the association between the word and the notion of relaxation, the greater the power of the cue word for the athlete. It has been recommended that the cue word should be paired at least 20 times a day with exhaling to build this skill over time (Payne, 2004). The use of an appropriate cue word is also often used as part of centering. It should also be noted that when using imagery techniques relaxation is also commonly used in combination. Whilst it is not the intention of the authors to outline every possible intervention paired with relaxation, it is hoped that the athlete's and the sport medicine professionals' attention is alerted to the possibilities of pairing each of the psychological intervention techniques from Chapters 5–9. When deciding on the most appropriate intervention or intervention package, the expertise of the professional working with the athlete, as well as the preference of the athlete should be taken into account (Payne, 2004). Techniques that appeal to an individual are more likely to gain their co-operation and result in more effective rehabilitation.

Relaxation techniques that can be beneficial during injury rehabilitation include PMR, breath control techniques and passive relaxation. To maximise rehabilitation, these techniques can be paired with other techniques such as functional self-talk and imagery.

Practical advice for sport medicine professionals when implementing relaxation techniques

Regardless of the relaxation technique employed, there are several prerequisites necessary to facilitate effective relaxation. These include educating the injured athlete, providing a suitable environment for the relaxation to take place, ensuring that there is an appropriate structure to the relaxation programme, measuring relaxation effectiveness and adopting appropriate relaxation techniques in accordance with the phase of rehabilitation.

Educating the athlete

Education is vital as a first step for any relaxation training (Rotella, 1982). The athlete should be educated about the purpose, the benefits and the reasons for the use of relaxation. The athlete should also be given opportunities to ask questions and share any apprehensions about the technique and these should be resolved with the athlete's best interests in mind. For example, the sport medicine professional might explain to the injured athlete that a relaxation technique may help them because it promotes blood supply to the injured site and blood has healing properties. They might also be informed that these techniques will give them a sense of being in control of their recovery. They do, however, need to be reminded when using PMR, for example, to take care on the tension phase when the injury location is being used and to only continue as long as they are pain free.

Providing a suitable environment for relaxation

Ensuring the environment is suitable for relaxation is also important. A quiet, comfortable atmosphere is considered more facilitative to relaxation (Crossman, 2001; Rotella, 1982; Taylor and Taylor, 1997). However, this is not always practical in a sport or rehabilitation setting. The athlete should be positioned comfortably (ideally lying down or seated in a chair). Particularly in the initial stages of learning, it is useful for the eyes to be closed and for the individual to concentrate on how their body feels and rid the mind of all other thoughts (Crossman, 2001).

Ensuring that there is an appropriate structure to the relaxation programme

Relaxation is also said to be most effective when integrated into the structure of daily sessions (for example, using ratio breathing during the times when pain is high; Taylor and Taylor, 1997). Relaxation is a skill and, like all other skills, it requires practice (Flint, 1998) and the ability to use these techniques is directly related to the amount of time spent practising them. It is also important that the athlete does not expect too much too soon.

Measuring relaxation effectiveness

It might also be useful to use physiological (heart rate, respiration rate, blood pressure) and psychological self-rating scales for assessing pain and anxiety reduction when using relaxation techniques. These measurements might help the sport medicine professional in determining the effectiveness of the technique and also help the injured athlete see the benefits of the technique too. Ending rehabilitation sessions with a relaxation session is also perceived as being beneficial, since it can be a rejuvenating experience following a painful and possibly unpleasant experience (Taylor and Taylor, 1997).

Using appropriate relaxation techniques during different phases of rehabilitation

As rehabilitation consists of three main phases (the injury phase, rehabilitation phase and return to sport phase; for more details see Chapter 10), ensuring the appropriateness of relaxation techniques in each phase is of importance. For example, during phase I, when pain is at its worst, using physical relaxation is important to help manage pain. In this phase, the sport medicine professional might teach an injured athlete deep breathing techniques and encourage the use of cue words that induce a state of relaxation (Walsh, 2011). During phase II, the focus might be to reduce the stress response to injury. By integrating relaxation techniques into rehabilitation, the athlete may be more able to manage their anxieties. In this phase, the pairing of relaxation with imagery can increase effort and persistence in rehabilitation, as well as continuing to be used to manage pain associated with rehabilitation exercises. In phase III, the athlete will be eager to return to training and competition and re-injury anxiety might be salient at this time (Walker and Thatcher, 2011). The ability to induce a state of relaxation is an important skill and should be emphasised in response to the increase of anxiety during this phase.

Conclusion

This chapter has introduced the importance of relaxation techniques in sport injury rehabilitation and outlined the types of relaxation techniques used in sport injury rehabilitation. The chapter then summarised the literature pertinent to use of relaxation techniques in sport injury rehabilitation and discussed the ways in which relaxation techniques can be combined with other psychological interventions. Moreover, the chapter provided practical advice to those working with injured athletes on how to maximise the use of relaxation techniques with injured athletes. Based on the evidence presented, a range of relaxation techniques can be of use for injured athletes during rehabilitation and on their return to training and competition. Relaxation can facilitate athletes' ability to manage and alleviate pain, to deal with stress and anxiety, and enhance physiological recovery.

CASE STUDY

Hari is a 21-year-old male international cricketer (right-hand batter, right-arm fast bowler), who has a torn anterior cruciate ligament. Hari is a bright prospect who is expected to fill in the vacancies created by the retirement of more experienced internationals. Before his injury, he became only the third Indian batsman to hit back-to-back centuries in one day internationals. Since sustaining his injury, Hari feels under pressure to return to his previous fitness and form as soon as possible and is finding being injured very frustrating. He has recently had reconstructive surgery and is experiencing high levels of anxiety and is feeling very stressed in response to the injury. He is frustrated at the limitations that the injury had imposed and feels very angry that the injury occurred at a time when he was in good form. He has stated that he feels very tight around the shoulders and jaw and did not feel this way before the injury.

When informed that he would be on crutches for at least six weeks and approximately six to eight months of further rehabilitation, he also described feeling his heart race and feeling sick. He feels that the injury is out of his control and that there is very little he can do to aid his rehabilitation.

—————— **?** ——————

1. Outline which relaxation techniques might be beneficial for Hari's recovery.
2. Outline how and why these relaxation techniques might be beneficial for Hari's recovery.
3. How might using a multiple intervention package, such as self-talk and progressive muscular relaxation, be useful to help Hari with his recovery?

References

Arvinen-Barrow, M., Hemmings, B., Weigand, D. A., Becker, C. A. and Booth, L. (2007) Views of chartered physiotherapists on the psychological content of their practice: A national follow-up survey in the United Kingdom. *Journal of Sport Rehabilitation*, 16, 111–21.

Baer, R. A. (2003) Mindfulness training as a clinical intervention: A conceptual and empirical review. *Clinical Psychology: Science and Practice*, 10, 125–43.

Beneka, A., Malliou, P., Bebetsos, E., Gioftsidou, A., Pafis, G. and Godolias, G. (2007) Appropriate counselling techniques for specific components of the rehabilitation plan: A review of the literature. *Physical Training,* August. Retrieved from http://ejmas.com/pt/ptframe.htm.

Benson, H. and Klipper, M. Z. (2000) *The Relaxation Response: Updated and expanded.* New York: Harper Collins.

Benson, H. and Proctor, W. (1984) *Beyond the Relaxation Response.* New York: Berkeley.

Bernier, M., Thienot, E., Codron, R. and Fournier, J. F. (2009) Mindfulness and acceptance approaches in sport performance. *Journal of Clinical Sports Psychology*, 4, 320–33.

Brown, K. W. and Ryan, R. M. (2003) The benefits of being present: Mindfulness and its role in psychological well-being. *Journal of Personality and Social Psychology*, 84, 822–48.

Caroll, D. and Seers, K. (1998) Relaxation for the relief of chronic pain: a systematic review. *Journal of Advanced Nursing*, 27, 476–87.

Christakou, A. and Lavallee, D. (2009) Rehabilitation from sports injuries: From theory to practice. *Perspectives in Public Health*, 129(3), 120–6.

Christakou, A. and Zervas, Y. (2007) The effectiveness of imagery on pain, edema, and range of motion in athletes with grade II ankle sprain. *Physical Therapy in Sport*, 8(3), 130–41.

Cottraux, J. (2007) *Thérapie Cognitive et Emotions: La troisième vague* [Cognitive Therapy and Emotions: The third wave]. Paris: Elsevier Masson.

Cousin, M. J. and Philips, G. D. (1985) Acute pain management. In M. J. Cousin and G. D. Philips (eds), *Clinics in Critical Care Medicine* (Volume 8). New York: Churchill Livingstone.

Crews, D. J. (1993) Self-regulation strategies in sport and exercise. In R. N. Singer, M. Murphy and L. K. Tennant (eds), *Handbook of Research on Sport Psychology*. New York: MacMillan, pp. 557–68.

Crossman, J. (2001) Managing thoughts, stress, and pain. In J. Crossman (ed.), *Coping with Sport Injuries: psychological strategies for rehabilitation*. New York: Oxford University Press, pp. 128–47.

Cupal, D. D. and Brewer, B. W. (2001) Effects of relaxation and guided imagery on knee strength, re-injury anxiety, and pain following anterior cruciate ligament reconstruction. *Rehabilitation Psychology*, 46(1), 28–43.

Dosil, J. (2006) *The Sport Psychologist's Handbook: A guide for sport-specific performance enhancement*. Chichester: Wiley & Sons.

Flint, F. A. (1998) Integrating sport psychology and sports medicine in research: The dilemmas. *Journal of Applied Sport Psychology*, 10, 83–102.

Flint, F. A. (2007) Modeling in injury rehabilitation: Seeing helps believing. In D. Pargman (ed.), *Psychological Bases of Sport Injuries*. Morgantown, WV: Fitness Information Technology, pp. 95–107.

Garcia, R. F., Villa, R. S., Cepeda, N. T., Cueto, E. G. and Montes, J. M. G. (2004) Efecto de la hipnosis y la terapia de aceptcion y compromiso (ACT) en la mejora de la fuerza fisica en piraguistas. *International Journal of Clinical and Health Psychology*, 4, 481–93.

Gardner, F. L. and Moore, Z. E. (2004) A Mindfulness–Acceptance–Commitment. MAC based approach to athletic performance enhancement: Theoretical considerations. *Behavior Therapy*, 35, 707–23.

Gardner, F. L. and Moore, Z. E. (2006) *Clinical Sport Psychology*. Champaign, IL.: Human Kinetics.

Green, L. B. and Bonura, K. B. (2007) The use of imagery in the rehabilitation of injured athletes. In D. Pargman (ed.), *Psychological Bases of Sport Injuries*, 3rd edn. Morgantown, WV: Fitness Information Technology, pp. 131–47.

Harwood, C. (1998) *Handling Pressure*. Leeds: The National Coaching Foundation.

Heaney, C. (2006) Physiotherapists' perceptions of sport psychology intervention in professional soccer. *International Journal of Sport and Exercise Psychology*, 4(1), 67–80.

Heil, J. (1993) A framework of psychological assessment. In J. Heil (ed.), *Psychology of Sport Injury*. Champaign, IL: Human Kinetics, pp. 73–87.

Hill, K. L. (2001) *Frameworks for Sport Psychologists*. Champaign, IL: Human Kinetics.

Jacobs, G. D. (2001) The physiology of mind–body interactions: The stress response and the relaxation response. *Journal of Alternative and Complementary Medicine*, 7, 583–92.

Jacobson, E. (1938) *Progressive Relaxation*. Chicago, IL: University of Chicago Press.

Jessup, B. A. and Gallegos, X. (1994) Relaxation and biofeedback. In P. D. Wall and R. Melzack (eds), *Textbook of Pain*. Oxford: Elsevier.

Kabat–Zinn, J. (1994) *Wherever You Go, There Are You: Mindfulness meditation in everyday life*. New York: Hyperion.

Keable, D. (1989) *The Management of Anxiety. A manual for therapists*. London: Churchill Livingstone.

Kee, Y. H. and Wang, C. K. J. (2008) Relationships between mindfulness, flow dispositions, and mental skills adoption: A cluster analytic approach. *Psychology of Sport and Exercise*, 9, 393–411.

Linton, S. J. (1994) Chronic back pain: Integrating psychological and physical therapy – An overview. *Behavioural Medicine*, 20, 101–4.

Ma, S. H. and Teasdale, J. D. (2004) Mindfulness-based cognitive therapy for depression: Replication and exploration of differential relapse prevention effects. *Journal of Consulting and Clinical Psychology*, 72, 31–40.

Mahoney, J. and Hanrahan, S. (2011) A brief educational intervention using acceptance and commitment therapy: Four injured athletes' experiences. *Journal of Clinical Sport Psychology*, 5, 252–73.

Manzoni, G. M., Pagnini, F., Castelnuovo, G. and Molinari, E. (2008) Relaxation training for anxiety: A ten-years systematic review with meta-analysis. *BCM Psychiatry*, 8, 41–52.

McCaffery, M. and Pasero, C. (1999) Assessment: Underlying complexities, misconceptions, and practical tools. In M. McCaffery and C. Pasero (eds), *Pain clinical manual*, 2nd edn. St. Louis, MI: Mosby, pp. 35–102.

McConnell, A. (2011) *Breathe Strong Perform Better*. Champaign, IL: Human Kinetics.

Moore, Z. E. (2009) Theoretical and empirical developments of the mindfulness–acceptance–commitment (MAC) approach to performance enhancement. *Journal of Clinical Sports Psychology*, 4, 291–302.

Naoi, A. and Ostrow, A. (2008) The effects of cognitive and relaxation interventions on injured athletes mood and pain during rehabilitation. *Athletic Insight*, 10(1). Retrieved from http://www.athleticinsight.com/Vol10Iss1/InterventionsInjury.htm.

Ost, L. G. (1988) Applied relaxation: Description of an effective coping technique. Scandinavian *Journal of Behavior Therapy*, 17, 83–96.

Owens, M. K. and Ehrenreich, D. (1991) Literature review of nonpharmacologic methods for the treatment of chronic pain. *Holistic Nursing Practice*, 6, 24–31.

Payne, S. (2004) Relaxation techniques. In G. S. Kolt and M. B. Andersen (eds), *Psychology in the Physical and Manual Therapies*. London: Churchill Livingstone, pp. 111–24.

Rotella, R. J. (1982) Psychological care of the injured athlete. In D. N. Kulund (ed.), *The injured athlete*. Philadelphia, PA: Lippincott, pp. 213–24.

Schultz, J. and Luthe, W. (1969) *Autogenic Methods*, 1. New York: Grune and Stratton.

Taylor, J. and Taylor, S. (1997) *Psychological Approaches to Sports Injury Rehabilitation*. Gaithersburg, MD: Aspen.

Taylor, J. and Taylor, S. (1998) Pain education and management in the rehabilitation from sports injury. *The Sport Psychologist*, 12, 68–88.

Wagman, D. and Khelifa, M. (1996) Psychological issues in sport injury rehabilitation: Current knowledge and practice. *Journal of Athletic Training*, 31(3), 257–61.

Walker, N. (2006) The meaning of sports injury and re-injury anxiety assessment and intervention (PhD thesis). University of Wales, Aberystwyth.

Walker, N. and Thatcher, J. (2011) The emotional response to athletic injury: Re-injury anxiety. In J. Thatcher, M. V. Jones and D. Lavallee (eds), *Coping and Emotion in Sport*, 2nd edn. New York: Routledge, pp. 235–59.

Walsh, A. E. (2011) The relaxation response: A strategy to address stress. *International Journal of Athletic Therapy and Training*, 16(2), 20–23.

Weinberg, R. S. and Gould, D. (2011) *Foundations of Sport and Exercise Psychology*. Champaign, IL: Human Kinetics.

Williams, J. M. and Andersen, M. B. (2007) Psychosocial antecedents of sport injury and interventions for risk reduction. In G. Tenenbaum and R. Eklund (eds), *Handbook of Sport Psychology*, 3rd edn. Hoboken, NJ: Wiley, pp. 379–403.

Yukelson, D. and Murphy, S. (1993) Psychological considerations in injury prevention. In P. A. F. H. Renstrom (ed.), *Sports Injuries: Basic principles of prevention and care*. Malden, MA: Blackwell Scientific Publications, pp. 321–33.

8

SELF-TALK IN SPORT INJURY REHABILITATION

Natalie Walker and Joanne Hudson

> *How you think affects how you perform and how you rehabilitate.*
> *(Phil, sport medicine professional)*

Introduction

It is understood that most athletes engage in some form of self-talk. The thoughts an injured athlete has and the things they say to themselves regarding their injury are proposed to influence their emotions, behaviours and recovery outcomes (Wiese-Bjornstal, Smith, Shaffer and Morrey, 1998). However, the extent, frequency, content and type of self-talk can vary depending on the situation and the individual (Zinsser, Bunker and Williams, 2006). For example, the level at which the athlete competes at and skill type have been suggested as moderators of self-talk use (Tod, Hardy and Oliver, 2011). This chapter outlines the role of self-talk in sport injury rehabilitation by: (a) initially outlining the concept of self-talk in the wider context of sport, (b) introducing the different types of self-talk used in sport, (c) describing the functions of these different types of self-talk, (d) discussing the use of self-talk during rehabilitation and finally concluding with (e) an outline of the process of self-talk use during rehabilitation.

The concept of self-talk

Based on considerable lack of clarity in the literature, it has been argued that a consensus was needed regarding an accepted definition of self-talk (Hardy, Jones and Gould, 1996). It was not until a decade later that such discussions began to take place (Hardy, 2006). A number of definitions of self-talk have since been proposed and are outlined in this section. According to Theodorakis, Weinberg, Natsis,

Douma, and Kazakas (2000), self-talk is 'what people say to themselves either out loud or as a small voice inside their head' (p. 254). This definition highlights two aspects of self-talk. That self-talk is expressed either overtly or covertly and that self-talk is composed of statements that are addressed to oneself and not to other people in the form of conversation. Hackford and Schwenkmezger (1993) proposed that self-talk is a 'dialogue [through which] the individual interprets feelings and perceptions, regulates and changes evaluations and convictions, and gives him/herself instructions and reinforcement' (p. 355). This definition offers both the notion that self-talk is concerned with making self-statements but also alludes to some of the uses of self-talk. We are therefore encouraged to define self-talk by the following guidelines: (a) it represents verbalisations or statements addressed to the self; (b) it is multidimensional in nature (for example, with frequency and valence properties); (c) it has interpretive elements associated with the content of statements employed; (d) it is dynamic; (e) it serves a function for the athlete (that is, it can be instructional and/or motivational; Hardy, 2006).

An overview of the types and functions of self-talk in sport

Overt/covert self-talk

As outlined previously, there is some discussion related to how the individual's self-statements are verbalised. At one end of the continuum, an individual might talk to themselves in a very overt fashion (externally verbalised statements), allowing others to hear what is said. At the other end of the continuum, covert self-talk is located, and is defined as verbalisations that are made by a small voice inside one's head or as an inner dialogue that cannot be heard by others. It is likely that an athlete engages in one or both types of self-talk. To date, research has yet to provide any conclusive evidence related to the effectiveness of overt compared with covert self-talk in the sport domain. However, based on similar principles in goal setting, where public goals are more effective than private goals (Kyllo and Landers, 1995), it might be expected that when statements are overt there could be some evaluation of the individual's performance related to those statements. Therefore, the individual might exert more effort to achieve the desired behaviours associated with overtly expressed statements.

Assigned and self-determined self-talk

There is also some discussion concerning the level to which an individual's self-talk statements are self-determined; that is, if their self-talk is 'assigned' or 'freely chosen' (Hardy, 2006). Assigned self-talk is where the individual has no self-determined control over the statements (that is, the statements are given to the athlete by someone else such as the sport medicine professional) and freely chosen self-talk is where the individual has completely determined their self-talk (that is, composed of their own statements). Despite limited examination of whether assigned or self-determined self-talk is more effective, it is more likely that an athlete would use self-talk that they determine themselves in performance settings (Hardy, 2006). It is also likely that, based on the principles of Deci and Ryan's (1985) cognitive evaluation theory, self-determined self-talk will offer more motivational benefits for the athlete (Hardy, 2006). Cognitive evaluation theory proposes that we have an innate desire to feel competent and self-determined and that an athlete's feeling of self-determination for their actions is related to their perceptions of choice. Hence, self-talk chosen by the athlete, theoretically, should have positive effects on their self-determined motivation.

> I've heard injured athletes I've worked with say some pretty awful and unhelpful things to themselves in my years as a physio. They can be their own worst enemy at times.
>
> (Phil, sport medicine professional)

Negative and positive self-talk

Traditionally, self-talk has been conceptualised as either positive or negative (Tod et al., 2011). Self-talk as a form of praise (Moran, 1996), that is used to keep one's focus of attention in the present has been commonly termed positive self-talk (Weinberg, 1988). However, self-talk, in the form of criticism (Moran, 1996) and which presents barriers to achieving because it is inappropriate, anxiety-provoking and/or irrational, has been called negative self-talk (Theodorakis et al., 2000). It is suggested that positive self-talk is performance facilitating whereas negative self-talk is performance debilitating (Hardy, 2006; Zinsser, Bunker and Williams, 2010). Following their systematic review of the literature, Tod et al. (2011) found evidence to confirm the proposed positive effect of self-talk on performance. No support was found, however, for an effect of negative self-talk. Sixty per cent of the research in their review indicated that positive self-talk was more beneficial for performance than negative self-talk and the remaining 40 per cent reported no performance differences between positive and negative self-talk (Tod et al., 2011).

Instructional and motivational self-talk

A more contemporary conceptualisation has been to view self-talk in relation to its function: instructional and/or motivational. The execution of precision-based tasks that require skill, timing and accuracy can be aided through instructional self-talk that increases attentional focus on relevant technical aspects of performance (Hatzigeorgiadis, Theodorakis and Zourbanos, 2004; Theodorakis et al., 2000). In contrast, motivational self-talk is suggested to be more effective than instructional self-talk for the execution of strength and endurance based tasks as this type of self-talk is used to increase effort, enhance confidence, and/or create positive moods (Tod *et al.*, 2011).

The two broad functions of self-talk (instructional and motivational) have been further refined into more specific functions. Instructional self-talk has been refined into two more specific instructional functions – *skills* and *general* related (Hardy, Gammage and Hall, 2001). Skill-specific instructions focus on the technique of a skill and might include statements such as 'keep the hands together'. Instructional general self-talk includes statements about strategies that are important for performance. For example, 'stay in second until the last bend'. With respect to motivational self-talk, this has been further refined into three more specific motivational functions – *arousal*, *mastery*, and *drive* (Hardy *et al.*, 2001). The motivational arousal function refers to the use of self-talk in psyching up, relaxing and controlling arousal. The motivational mastery function relates to mental toughness, focus of attention, confidence and mental preparation. The motivational drive function is concerned with goal achievement and consequently is associated with maintaining or increasing drive and effort.

The findings from Tod *et al.*'s (2011) systematic literature review suggest that both instructional and motivational self-talk had a positive effect on precision-based tasks. Similarly, they reported that instructional and motivational self-talk had a positive effect on gross motor-skill performance (Tod *et al.*, 2011). They concluded therefore that, contrary to what has previously been suggested, instructional self-talk was not consistently more effective than motivational self-talk for the execution of precision-based tasks and that motivational self-talk was not more effective than instructional self-talk for gross motor-skill tasks (Tod *et al.*, 2011).

A conceptual framework was proposed by Hardy, Oliver, and Tod (2009) to explain factors which they believe mediate the self-talk performance relationship (Table 8.1). This framework highlights why simple relationships between self-talk and performance do not exist and why they are not consistent. It also allows practitioners to use self-talk interventions more effectively in practice.

It should be noted that more research is needed on this conceptual framework of self-talk. Similarly, more research is needed on self-talk in injury rehabilitation. The following section provides a brief summary of the key studies on self-talk in rehabilitation to date.

Key research from the self-talk literature in sport injury rehabilitation

A limited amount of empirical research has investigated the use of psychological intervention strategies in a sport injury context (Evans, Mitchell and Jones, 2006). The literature that does exist suggests that self-talk is useful for joint restoration, muscular strengthening and rehearsing sport-related skills whilst injured (Beneka *et al.*, 2007). Ievleva and Orlick (1991) were the first authors to study the impact of psychological interventions on athletes' recovery from sport injury. In their retrospective study with rehabilitated athletes, they reported a link between recovery

TABLE 8.1 A conceptual framework of self-talk

Self-talk factor	Influence on performance
Cognitive	Athletes adopt self-talk for a variety of attention-based outcomes (e.g. concentration) thus manipulating self-talk may also be useful to alter attentional foci.
Motivational	The use of self-talk is thought to affect the persistence or long-term goal commitment of an individual via self-talk acting as an antecedent to self-efficacy (Tod et al., 2011).
Behavioural	There is evidence of improvements in technique with the use of self-talk (Hardy et al., 2009). During the early phases of learning, it has been proposed that novices may 'talk' themselves through movements, resulting in changes in movement patterns or technical execution which could then underlie performance improvements (Hardy et al., 2011).
Affective	There is a wealth of literature suggesting a link between cognitive content and affect and, in turn, affect and performance. For example, there is widespread support that self-talk might influence anxiety in sporting performance (e.g. Maynard et al., 1995).

Source: Hardy et al. (2009)

time and the use of positive self-talk. The fast healers reported greater use of goal setting, imagery and self-talk than their slower healing counterparts. The qualitative findings identified that the fast-healing athletes had a tendency to be more positive than the slower healers. These findings show some support for an athlete's ability to influence and control their thoughts during the injury and rehabilitation process and the positive use of self-talk during rehabilitation.

In a series of studies exploring the use of coping strategies by injured athletes, further support for the benefits of self-talk were suggested (Gould, Eklund and Jackson, 1993). Eighty per cent of Olympic wrestlers who were interviewed in this study stated that they used thought control strategies as a means of coping with their injuries. Rational thinking and self-talk were also reported as the most popular coping strategies employed by injured national championship-level figure skaters in a study by Gould, Finch, and Jackson (1993). Similar findings were reported by Gould, Udry, Bridges, and Beck (1997) in relation to exploring coping with season-ending injuries.

Positive self-talk has also been found to generate positive emotions that are associated with an enhanced quality of rehabilitation (Udry, Gould, Bridges and Beck, 1997). Rock and Jones (2002) provided support for the use of reframing an athlete's cognitions as part of the rehabilitation process during counselling sessions. More specifically, it was concluded that engaging in such interventions during rehabilitation could have a positive effect on athletes' psychological wellbeing, particularly during setbacks in the recovery process (Rock and Jones, 2002).

In her doctoral thesis, Walker (2006) also provided support for the use of reframing paired with progressive muscular relaxation during rehabilitation from sport injury. She measured injured athletes' re-injury anxiety using the re-injury anxiety inventory (RIAI; Walker, Thatcher and Lavallee, 2010). Using a multiple-baseline design, the players' re-injury anxieties were explored before and after the introduction of the intervention. Following the introduction of the intervention, there was a quick reduction in trend, mean and level for both re-injury anxiety related to rehabilitation (RIA-R) and re-injury anxiety related to returning to training/competition (RIA-RE). Social validation results also showed that the participants perceived positive changes in re-injury anxieties as a consequence of using the intervention.

The most recent published investigation exploring the use of self-talk for injured athletes was conducted by Naoi and Ostrow (2008). A single-subject design was employed, similar to that adopted by Walker (2006), and changes in mood and pain responses were measured via standardised psychological instruments (Naoi and Ostrow, 2008). Three of the five injured athletes showed an improvement in mood during the intervention phase compared with the baseline phase but all athletes reported that the intervention was an aid to their physical and psychological recovery.

Self-talk techniques in sport injury rehabilitation

Positive self-talk has generally been advocated as being more useful than negative self-talk (Zinsser et al., 2010); hence, it has been proposed that athletes should be helped to reduce their use of negative self-talk and increase their use of more positive self-talk. However, as previously outlined, Tod et al. (2011) suggest that, despite support for the use of positive self-talk compared with no self-talk, an inconsistent effect has been detected for the possible benefits of positive self-talk over the use of negative self-talk. Hamilton, Scott, and MacDougall (2007) describe negative self-talk as 'challenging' self-talk in some circumstances and for some athletes rather than negative self-talk. Therefore, the interpretation of the content of self-talk is more important than the actual type of self-talk itself (that is, positive or negative; Hamilton et al., 2007). For example, following an inappropriate behaviour (for example, missing a rehabilitation session) an athlete might give themselves a 'talking to' (for instance, 'You idiot! This will not help you') and hence be motivated not to repeat the same behaviour in the future. This type of self-talk (negative statements) might only be harmful to some athletes but for others it might actually be facilitative (Goodhart, 1986; Van Raalte, Cornelius, Brewer and Hatten, 2000). For this reason, from here onwards we use the term 'functional self-talk' in this chapter. The following section outlines the use of thought stopping and reframing as two potential techniques for encouraging functional self-talk in rehabilitation.

Thought stopping

Thought stopping has been proposed to be useful by some authors (for example, Bull, Albinson and Shambrook, 1996) to initially stop an inappropriate thought and then allow a more functional thought to be used in its place. Thought stopping has been advocated as a deliberate self-talk technique to direct sport-related thinking (Zinsser *et al.*, 2006).

Thought-stopping steps

1. Increase the athlete's awareness of the inappropriate self-talk they are using. For example, they might keep paperclips in one pocket and transfer a paperclip to the opposite pocket on each use of inappropriate self-talk in rehabilitation (Owens and Bunker, 1989). At the end of the session, the athlete can see how many paperclips they have in the 'inappropriate self-talk' pocket, increasing their awareness of its use.

2. Once the injured athlete is aware of their use of inappropriate self-talk, the second step is to use a trigger to stop the thoughts/talk (cue word, image or action). For example, an athlete might say 'wait' or might visualise an image of a stop sign or snap their fingers as a trigger to stop their inappropriate self-talk statements.

3. Finally, a more functional self-talk statement is then used to replace the previous inappropriate self-talk. This final step is important because, when thought-stopping techniques are used on their own without supplementary techniques, this is likely to exacerbate the problem of inappropriate self-talk.

(Hardy et al., *2009)*

Some self-talk that is perceived as negative might in fact be challenging, and therefore motivational, and might not need to be stopped or changed. The key for the practitioner is to initially explore the athlete's interpretation of their self-talk.

Reframing technique

A common response to injury is anxiety (for example, anxieties related to pain experienced, lengthy rehabilitation anxieties, the loss of a starting place and changes to daily routines, performance outcome anxieties, pre and/or post-operative anxiety, fitness demands and returning to peak performance anxiety and re-injury anxiety). When faced with a potentially anxiety-provoking situation, there is a need to challenge these appraisals. This can be achieved via modifying the athlete's thoughts and self-statements associated with the situation, a technique called reframing. Here the event or behaviour stays the same but the athlete's appraisal is changed (Jones, 2003).

There is a substantial amount of anecdotal evidence reporting the benefits of reframing in the field of sport and exercise psychology (see, for example, Bull *et al.*, 1996; Porter, 2003; Syer and Connolly, 1998). However, there appears to be substantially more empirical research using the reframing technique in counselling psychology.

- The key to reframing begins with awareness of the nature of the self-talk/thought. The first stage is, therefore, developing awareness of current thoughts/talk.
- Once the inappropriate cognitions are exposed, the athlete can challenge them by reframing the appraisal to a more functional counter response. The reframing technique involves reappraisal of a situation to programme the subconscious for success and lay the foundations for future progress and change (Hill, 2001). Altering the appraisal of an event or situation effects a change in the way feelings and emotions are attached to that situation (Hill, 2001). As a result of the change, behaviour and responses will change.

An injured athlete's thoughts and statements before, during and after injury, including rehabilitation, have been shown to be a critical element of the psychological response to injury (see Chapters 2 and 3). It is reported that injured athletes often engage in inappropriate self-talk and that this is often counterproductive. The literature outlined earlier discusses evidence that self-talk is a psychological intervention that is useful for aiding recovery from an athletic injury. By challenging an injured athlete's inappropriate thoughts and statements practitioners can reduce the potential detrimental impact that they can have on emotions, rehabilitation compliance and adherence, and recovery outcomes. In chapter 10, the authors outline three phases of rehabilitation. Table 8.2 outlines examples of the use of reframing during these three phases.

It is important to offer functional self-talk, or indeed any intervention, early in rehabilitation to allow the athlete time to become familiar with it (Walker, 2006).

Functional self-talk might be particularly useful at phase III for focusing the injured athlete on thoughts associated with successfully performing the skills they need for their sport.

Using self-affirming functional self-talk to build confidence for the return to training and competition is also critical during rehabilitation.

TABLE 8.2 Reframing during the three phases of rehabilitation

Phase of rehabilitation	Injury experience	Self-talk	Reframed self-talk
I	Unhelpful negative thoughts about injury severity; the significance of the injury to their future; blame themselves for injury onset; struggling to cope with the pain of the injury; concerned about the prospect of a difficult and possibly long rehabilitation process	'This is agony! I can't believe I went in for that tackle.'	'I can handle this I'm tough. I am not the only person ever to be injured. The pain prevents me from doing more damage.'
II	Loss of motivation; coping with difficult and/or lengthy rehabilitation; anxieties about becoming re-injured during rehabilitation	'I can't go on the board. I can't balance. I'm going to fall off and twist it again.'	'I've balanced on an uneven surface. The board is no different. It's just the same, I can do it!'
III	Anxieties and doubts about their return to training and competition	'It's not strong enough. I need more rehab before testing it in training.'	'It has been tested throughout rehabilitation and it has survived. It is ready.'

Functional self-talk in sport injury rehabilitation

The types and functions of self-talk outlined in the opening of this chapter are also appropriate in the context of injury rehabilitation. An injured athlete is likely to engage in some inappropriate self-talk at some period of their injury experience. For example, they might say, 'I'm never going to recover from this injury'. They may also engage in more functional self-talk; for example, when struggling with motivation during rehabilitation they might say, 'You can do this! Only four more reps!' It could be expected that a mixture of both positive and negative self-talk said both overtly and/or covertly are used by an injured athlete throughout their rehabilitation. Whilst not all negative self-talk is *always* debilitative, as outlined earlier, athletes should try to engage in more functional self-talk because it is likely to be more facilitative in rehabilitation settings.

> *I don't care whether the athlete says things about their recovery out loud or to themselves. For me the importance is what they are saying. They have to believe seeing their injury and recovery in a more positive light is far better than beating themselves up. Some find positive things to say to themselves and others need some help when they say really bad things to see a more positive view to the situation. I can help them with that, I like to challenge what they are thinking and saying about their injury.*
>
> *(Sally, sport medicine professional)*

The sport medicine professional might encourage an injured athlete to engage in many types of functional self-talk for a variety of purposes (to motivate or to instruct). Table 8.3 demonstrates some example self-talk statements for the five different functions of self-talk.

TABLE 8.3 Examples of self-talk serving different functions in injury rehabilitation

Type of self-talk	Example
Instructional:	
Skills	'Keep the heel flat'
Strategy	'This is boring but small steps lead to recovery'
Motivational:	
Arousal	'Come on! You can do this.'
	'Stay relaxed, breathe slow.'
Mastery	'The ankle is strong like a brick, I'm ready!'
Drive	'Push on, only 3 more reps!'

Self-determined and assigned self-talk in sport injury rehabilitation

It might also be appropriate for the sport medicine professional to consider the implications of assigning an athlete self-talk statements. Where possible an athlete should determine their own statements. However, where an athlete's appraisals of their injury are debilitative they may need help in challenging their appraisals and further assistance in restructuring their self-talk so that it is more functional. It would be unrealistic to expect the athlete engaging in inappropriate self-talk to come up with restructured self-talk independently and spontaneously. It might not be wise, however, to assign the athlete new self-talk statements. Collaborating with the athlete is vital in this instance. To do this, a practitioner might use the technique of reframing and encourage the athlete to record their negative thoughts regarding their injury and explore them during rehabilitation sessions, challenging the thoughts the athlete has. An awareness of self-talk patterns is often seen as the most difficult part of self-talk techniques (Taylor and Taylor, 1997). After raising the athlete's awareness, the sport medicine professional would encourage the athlete to reframe these statements into more personal functional affirmations (Porter, 2003). It is crucial that the reframed statements are true or, at least, probable and realistic (Crossman, 2001).The athlete might also be encouraged to destroy the debilitative statements and place them in a waste bin (Porter, 2003) and to re-read the restructured functional affirmations daily, reframing any debilitating thoughts that arise. For example, the injured athlete might say 'I can't attack the ball anymore because it [head injury] will happen again'.They might be helped to challenge this appraisal and restructure the statement to, 'I can attack the ball, I've done it loads before, and can make a difference to this game'.

> Self-talk might be self-determined and this is usually what we would encourage. However, some support and assistance might be needed to help injured athletes to develop functional self-talk statements.

Intervention efficacy beliefs

It is suggested that a belief or expectancy about intervention effectiveness may be a precondition for it to be effective (see, for example, Oikawa, 2004). It would be ineffective to use self-talk techniques with an injured athlete who does not expect them to be useful for their injury rehabilitation. It is also important to note that the sport medicine professional's belief in the intervention is also likely to be a precondition for self-talk to be effective. Thus, practitioners need to be aware of this before employing any intervention in rehabilitation. In addition, the working alliance or collaborative relationship between the sport medicine professional and the injured athlete may influence the athlete's belief in and willingness to use self-talk (see Tod and Andersen, 2005).

Conclusion

Self-talk can have a number of functions (such as to instruct on skill execution and skill strategy, to regulate arousal, focus attention and concentration and to aid in goal attainment). Its interpretation by the user is a critical determinant of outcomes of its use (not all negative self-talk has a negative consequence). Research supports the use of self-talk in sport generally but its use with injured athletes has less support currently. Early discussions from the small research base suggest that it can be used throughout rehabilitation for reducing recovery time, enhancing coping resources and the perception of quality of rehabilitation, improving joint restoration, increasing muscular strength, enhancing positive mood state and psychological wellbeing, reducing re-injury anxieties and allowing the athlete to rehearse sport-related skills whilst injured. However, further research is needed and should explore the athlete's experiences of using self-talk as part of the rehabilitation process.

Furthermore, the different motivational and cognitive functions of self-talk (as identified by Hardy *et al.*, 2001) should be explored in the sport injury rehabilitation setting.

CASE STUDY

Max is a 23-year-old martial artist who competes in Ju-Jitsu and has been engaging in rehabilitation after sustaining a grade II anterior talofibular ligament (ATFL) injury he suffered in training six weeks ago, after jumping to complete a spinning roundhouse kick and landing awkwardly on the mat. He has passed through the required three phases of rehabilitation (i.e., phase I the acute phase, phase II the rehabilitative phase, and phase III the functional phase) and he is approaching re-entry to training. However, he is demonstrating some anxieties about re-injury when he discusses his imminent return to sport. Sally, the sport medicine professional responsible for Max's care, has assured Max that he is physically rehabilitated from his injury and, based on the discussions between Sally and Max about his anxieties, she has asked Max to complete the RIAI (Walker *et al.*, 2010). His re-injury anxiety score regarding rehabilitation was 0 (indicating an absence of re-injury anxiety). However, his re-injury anxiety score regarding the return to training and competition was 40, indicating high re-injury anxieties in these environments (a maximum score of 45 is possible on this scale). Max has expressed his doubts to Sally, 'I am going to set myself up for a jump and it's just going to go again, I know it!' and has questioned, 'What if he blocks it [opposition] and that's enough to set me back to square one?' and 'A sharp change of direction or a sweep to it and what if it happens again?'. Although Sally has informed Max that he is ready to return to training, he responded, 'I'm not convinced it's ready, I need to put it to the test more. I might just tape it to give it added strength'. He has also made claims related to a perceived long-term weakness in the injured site. He said, 'I've just got this feeling it's always going to be weak now and that's going to play on my mind before competing'. More recently, he has informed Sally that his anxieties about becoming re-injured in training or competition have caused him to feel tense and that his breathing and heart rate increase when he thinks about the possibility of re-injury.

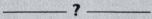

1. With reference to the integrated model of psychological response to sport injury and rehabilitation process outlined in Chapter 3 (Wiese-Bjornstal *et al.*, 1998), how might the technique of reframing reduce Max's re-injury anxieties?
2. How might using a multiple intervention package, such as reframing and progressive muscular relaxation, be useful to help Max with his holistic return to ju-jitsu training and competition?

3. Using the suggestions in this chapter, outline the procedure you would take when using reframing with Max.
4. Using the quotes from the case study, reframe the statements into more personal functional statements that Max might consider using.

References

Beneka, A., Malliou, P., Bebetsos, E., Gioftsidou, A., Pafis, G. and Godolias, G. (2007). Appropriate counselling techniques for specific components of the rehabilitation plan: A review of the literature. *Physical Training*. Retrieved from http://ejmas.com/pt/ptframe.htm.

Bull, S., Albinson, J. G. and Shambrook, C. J. (1996) *The Mental Game Plan: Getting psyched for sport*. Eastbourne: Sports Dynamics.

Crossman, J. (2001) Managing thoughts, stress, and pain. In J. Crossman (ed.), *Coping with Sport Injuries: Psychological strategies for rehabilitation*. New York: Oxford University Press, pp. 128–47.

Deci, E. L. and Ryan, R. M. (1985) *Intrinsic Motivation and Self-determination in Human Behavior*. New York: Plenum.

Evans, L., Mitchell, I. D. and Jones, S. (2006) Psychological responses to sport injury: A review of current research. In S. Hanton and S. D. Mellalieu (eds), *Literature Reviews in Sport Psychology*. New York: Nova Science, pp. 289–319.

Goodhart, D. E. (1986) The effects of positive and negative thinking on performance in an achievement situation. *Journal of Personality and Social Psychology*, 3, 219–36.

Gould, D., Eklund, R. C. and Jackson, S. A. (1993) Coping strategies used by US Olympic wrestlers *Research Quarterly for Exercise and Sport*, 64, 83–93.

Gould, D., Finch, L. M. and Jackson, S. A. (1993) Coping strategies used by national champion figure skaters. *Research Quarterly for Exercise and Sport*, 64(4), 453–68.

Gould, D., Udry, E., Bridges, D. and Beck, L. (1997) Coping with season-ending injuries. *The Sport Psychologist*, 11, 379–99.

Hackford, D. and Schwenkmezger, P. (1993) Anxiety. In R. N. Singer, M. Murphy and L. K. Tennant (eds), *Handbook of Research on Sport Psychology*. New York: Macmillan, pp. 328–64.

Hamilton, R. A., Scott, D. and MacDougall, M. P. (2007) Assessing the effectiveness of self-talk interventions on endurance performance. *Journal of Applied Sport Psychology*, 19, 226–39.

Hardy, J. (2006) Speaking clearly: A critical review of the self-talk literature. *Psychology of Sport & Exercise*, 7, 81–97.

Hardy, J., Gammage, K. L. and Hall, C. R. (2001) A descriptive study of athlete self-talk. *The Sport Psychologist*, 15, 306–18.

Hardy, L., Jones, G. and Gould, D. (1996) Understanding psychological preparation for sport: Theory and practice of elite performers. Chichester: John Wiley & Sons.

Hardy, J., Oliver, E. and Tod, D. (2009) A framework for the study and application of self-talk within sport. In S. D. Mellalieu and S. Hanton (eds), *Advances in Applied Sport Psychology: A review*. London: Routledge, pp. 37–74.

Hatzigeorgiadis, A., Theodorakis, Y. and Zourbanos, N. (2004) Self-talk in the swimming pool: The effects of self-talk on thought content and performance on water-polo tasks. *Journal of Applied Sport Psychology*, 16, 138–50.

Hill, K. L. (2001) *Frameworks for Sport Psychologists*. Champaign, IL: Human Kinetics.

Ievleva, L. and Orlick, T. (1991) Mental links to enhanced healing: An exploratory study. *The Sport Psychologist*, 5, 25–40.

Jones, M. V. (2003) Controlling emotions in sport *The Sport Psychologist*, 17, 471–86.

Kyllo, L. B. and Landers, D. M. (1995) Goal setting in sport and exercise: A research synthesis to resolve the controversy. *Journal of Sport & Exercise Psychology*, 17, 117–37.

Moran, A. P. (1996) *The Psychology of Concentration in Sport Performers*. East Sussex: Psychology Press.

Naoi, A. and Ostrow, A. (2008) The effects of cognitive and relaxation interventions on injured athletes mood and pain during rehabilitation. *Athletic Insight*, 10(1). Retrieved from http://www.athleticinsight.com/Vol10Iss1/InterventionsInjury.htm

Oikawa, M. (2004) Does addictive distraction affect the relationship between the cognition of distraction effectiveness and depression? *Japanese Journal of Educational Psychology*, 52, 287–97.

Owens, D. D. and Bunker, L. K. (1989) *Golf: Steps to Success*. Champaign, IL, Leisure Press.

Porter, K. (2003) *The Mental Athlete*. Champaign, IL: Human Kinetics.

Rock, J. A. and Jones, M. V. (2002) A preliminary investigation into the use of counseling skills in support of rehabilitation from sport injury. *Journal of Sport Rehabilitation*, 11, 284–304.

Syer, J. and Connolly, C. (1998) *Sporting Body, Sporting Mind*. London: Simon & Schuster.

Taylor, J. and Taylor, S. (1997) *Psychological Approaches to Sports Injury Rehabilitation*. Gaithersburg, MD: Aspen.

Theodorakis, Y., Weinberg, R., Natsis, P., Douma, I. and Kazakas, P. (2000) The effects of motivational versus instructional self-talk on improving motor performance. *The Sport Psychologist*, 14, 253–71.

Tod, D. and Andersen, M. B. (2005) Success in sport psych: Effective sport psychologists. In S. Murphy (ed.), *The Sport Psych Handbook*. Champaign, IL: Human Kinetics, pp. 305–14.

Tod, D., Hardy, J. and Oliver, E. (2011) Effects of self-talk: A systematic literature review. *Journal of Sport and Exercise Psychology*, 33, 666–87.

Udry, E., Gould, D., Bridges, D. and Beck, L. (1997) Down but not out: Athlete responses to season-ending injuries. *Journal of Sport & Exercise Psychology*, 19, 229–48.

Van Raalte, J. L., Cornelius, A. E., Brewer, B. W. and Hatten, S. J. (2000) The antecedents and consequences of self-talk in competitive tennis. *Journal of Sport & Exercise Psychology*, 22, 345–56.

Walker, N. (2006) *The Meaning of Sports Injury and Re-injury Anxiety Assessment and Intervention*. (Doctoral dissertation). University of Wales, Aberystwyth.

Walker, N., Thatcher, J. and Lavallee, D. (2010) A preliminary development of the re-injury anxiety inventory (RIAI). *Physical Therapy in Sport*, 11(1), 23–9.

Weinberg, R. S. (1988) *The Mental Advantage: Developing your psychological skills in tennis*. Champaign, IL: Human Kinetics.

Wiese-Bjornstal, D. M., Smith, A. M., Shaffer, S. M. and Morrey, M. A. (1998) An integrated model of response to sport injury: Psychological and sociological dynamics. *Journal of Applied Sport Psychology*, 10, 46–69.

Zinsser, N., Bunker, L. and Williams, J. M. (2006) Cognitive techniques for building confidence and enhancing performance. In J. M. Williams (ed.), *Applied Sport Psychology: Personal growth to peak performance*, 5th edn. New York: McGraw-Hill, pp. 349–81.

Zinsser, N., Bunker, L. and Williams, J. M. (2010) Cognitive techniques for building confidence and enhancing performance. In J. M. Williams (ed.), *Applied Sport Psychology: Personal growth to peak performance*, 6th edn. Boston: McGraw-Hill, pp. 305–33.

9

SOCIAL SUPPORT IN SPORT INJURY REHABILITATION

Monna Arvinen-Barrow and Stephen Pack

Introduction

Social support has been one of the most rigorously and frequently researched psychosocial resources (Thoits, 1995). The notion that people feel the need to be associated with others who provide love, warmth, social ties and a sense of belonging has long been considered as an emotionally satisfying aspect of life. Indeed, many philosophers have discussed the social needs of people and psychologists have postulated needs for social caring and nurture (Fromm, 1955; Litwak and Szelenyi, 1969; Maslow, 1954, 1968). It has also been suggested that social support mediates the stress–health link, enabling individuals to better cope with stressful events, thereby reducing the likelihood that stress will lead to ill health (Sarason, Sarason and Gurung, 1997). A great deal of evidence exists regarding the availability of social support and the reduced risks of mental and physical illness (for example, Berkman, 1984; Cohen and Wills, 1985; Thoits, 1995).

In sporting contexts, social support has been identified as a useful coping resource when dealing with a variety of stressors (such as performance pressures, relationship problems, unexpected disruption to performance routines and depression arising from unfulfilled expectations; Gould, Finch and Jackson, 1993). Similarly, high levels of particular types of social support have been linked to the maintenance of flow states (Rees and Hardy, 2004), as well as direct and indirect reductions in the effects of stress consequently enhancing self-confidence (Rees and Freeman, 2007). Research has also demonstrated social support as beneficial to athletes when dealing with sport related burnout (Rees, 2007). Sarason, Sarason and Pierce (1990) also proposed social support as having a direct influence on performance, a notion which, for example, has recently received empirical support in tennis (Freeman and Rees, 2009; Rees and Freeman, 2010; Rees and Hardy, 2004; Rees, Hardy and Freeman, 2007).

Despite many athletes preferring to 'go it alone' (Hardy, Jones and Gould, 1996: 234), research literature seems to support the importance of social support provision, particularly during 'times of need' (Rees, 2007: 224); such as when an athlete becomes injured. Indeed, within the literature related to sport-related injury, social support has been proposed as being integral to the coping process and therefore has been considered as a beneficial adjunct within the rehabilitation process (Bianco, 2001; Podlog and Eklund, 2007a; Rotella and Heyman, 1993; Weiss and Troxel, 1986). This chapter discusses how social support might be applied within sport injury rehabilitation. Specifically, the chapter: (a) introduces existing concept definitions and purposes of social support within the injury context; (b) describes the mechanisms of social support; (c) introduces different types of social support that might be beneficial in sport injury rehabilitation; (d) discusses a range of potential sources of social support in sport injury rehabilitation; (e) outlines the process of providing social support in sport injury rehabilitation; and (f) highlights some issues to consider when providing social support to injured athletes.

Social support in rehabilitation: concept definitions and purpose

Within the sport context, social support has received a high level of research attention, yet there is currently little consensus with regard to defining it as a concept. However, proposed definitions have included 'knowing that one is loved and that others will do all they can when a problem arises' (Sarason *et al.*, 1990: 119). Specifically relating to the injury context, social support has been defined as a 'form of interpersonal connectedness which encourages the constructive expression of feelings, provides reassurance in times of doubt, and leads to improved communication and understanding' (Heil, 1993a: 145). Rees (2007) also described social support as a multifaceted process in which an athlete is aided by the existence of a caring and supportive network, as well as by their perception of other people's availability to provide help in times of need and by the actual receipt of support.

These definitions appear to centre upon a common theme with regard to people acting as a provider of resources when needed. In succinct terms, social support might be considered a coping resource; a social 'fund' from which people may draw when dealing with stressors (Thoits, 1995). Moreover, it has been argued that the primary purpose of social support during injury rehabilitation is to afford an athlete a sense of belonging and assurance, which might help to convey in real terms that they are not isolated in their experience of injury, and instead have a support network readily available to assist them in the rehabilitation process (Taylor and Taylor, 1997).

Mechanisms of social support

It is commonly accepted that social support influences injury rehabilitation by impacting on an individual's response to the injury process; thus, it is appropriate to discuss the mechanisms of social support acknowledged within the integrated model of psychological response to sport injury and rehabilitation process (Wiese-Bjornstal, Smith, Shaffer and Morrey, 1998) as outlined in Chapter 3. This model highlights social support as a situational factor affecting an injured athlete's cognitive appraisal of their injury, which in turn may influence their emotional and/or behavioural responses to the injury. In addition, engagement (or lack of engagement) with social support has been highlighted as a behavioural response to injury, which in turn might also influence an athlete's cognitive appraisal and/or emotional response to the injury (Wiese-Bjornstal *et al.*, 1998; for more details on the model, see Chapter 3).

To date, it is thought that social support facilitates injury rehabilitation through two mechanisms: by 'buffering' athletes from harmful effects of injury related stressors and by directly influencing the rehabilitation process without any association with stress (Mitchell, Neil, Wadey and Hanton, 2007; Rees, 2007) (Figure 9.1). Thus, the stress-buffering model proposes that high levels of support can provide a 'shield' and an indirect support mechanism against potential negative effects of injury, such as unrealistic/negative cognitive appraisal (for example, unrealistic rate of recovery expectations or decreased self-perception), undesired emotional responses (for example, feelings of depression or frustration and poor emotional coping skills) and undesired behavioural responses (for example, lack of rehabilitation adherence, substance abuse and malingering), each having been found to have a negative effect on overall recovery outcomes of injury. Consequently, the stress-buffering model also assumes that social support is not relevant to those who do not perceive their situation (that is, the injury) as stressful.

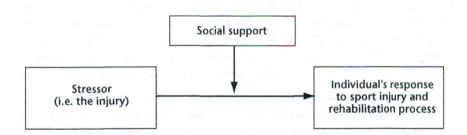

FIGURE 9.1   The stress-buffering effect model of social support adapted to sport injury settings

Source: adapted from Rees, 2007

In contrast, the main effect model proposes that social support can directly influence an individual's response to the injury and rehabilitation process (e.g., how an individual appraises the injury situation cognitively, emotionally, and behaviourally) (Figure 9.2). That is, having a supportive network offers the potential to increase positive affect, therefore increasing the likelihood of an athlete being more realistic about the rate of perceived recovery (cognitive appraisal), and subsequently

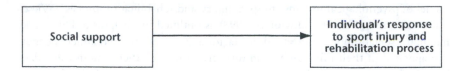

FIGURE 9.2 The main effects model of social support adapted to sport injury settings
Source: adapted from Rees, 2007

experiencing decreased levels of frustration and a more positive attitude towards rehabilitation (emotional response), leading to the potential for enhanced treatment compliance and rehabilitation adherence (behavioural response).

Whilst each model describes different causal explanations regarding how social support works, the two are considered as complementary (Bianco and Eklund, 2001). For example, an athlete may view injury as stress-provoking and, based upon the number of personal and situational factors (such as type/severity of injury and the rehabilitation environment) social support might help both directly and indirectly. Having assistance with everyday life chores (for example, food preparation) might directly impact athletes' responses to the injury and rehabilitation process by reducing potential daily hassles. Such support can also enable athletes to avoid unnecessary (potentially harmful) physical movement and thus directly impact the rate of physical recovery and recovery outcome. Similarly, having a supportive sport medicine professional to work with can also help athletes to approach the rehabilitation process with a more positive outlook, thus reducing the level of stress. In contrast, a lack of tangible day-to-day support might increase the stress felt by athletes. Therefore, not only is it important to understand how social support works during rehabilitation but also to understand what types of social support can be beneficial to athletes during the rehabilitation and recovery process.

Social support is a form of resource provision, arises from interpersonal connections, and its presence is consistently linked to beneficial health outcomes. For example, social support might 'buffer' injured athletes from potentially harmful effects of stress, directly influence appraisal of their injury in a helpful manner and aid the management of emotional and behavioural responses during the injury and rehabilitation process.

Types of social support

Existing literature generally considers social support as a multidimensional construct (Rees and Hardy, 2000). However, there is an ongoing disagreement regarding how many dimensions (or types of support) social support might comprise (Cutrona and Russell, 1990). Thus far, based on the works of Pines,

Aronson, and Kafry (1981), Hardy and Grace (1991, 1993) and Udry (1997, 2002) five distinct types of social support are considered as beneficial during sport injury rehabilitation: (1) emotional support, (2) technical support, (3) informational support, (4) tangible support and (5) motivational support. These can be further subdivided into more specific types of support: esteem support, listening support, emotional support, emotional challenge support, shared social reality support, technical appreciation support, technical challenge support, personal assistance support and material assistance support (Table 9.1).

As demonstrated above, there are a number of, often overlapping, types of social support that are said to be applicable to the sport injury context. Depending on the athlete and their personal situation, different types of support may be appropriate for different phases of rehabilitation (for more details on rehabilitation phases, see Chapter 10). For example, an athlete in phase I (reaction to injury) is often mostly concerned about the pain they are experiencing. Thus the provision of listening and emotional support, and possibly material assistance, might be most appropriate. During phase II (reaction to rehabilitation), an athlete is more likely to benefit from emotional challenge, technical appreciation and challenge support, as well as motivational support to help sustain/or increase motivation, rehabilitation adherence and/or treatment compliance. During phase III (reaction to return to play), esteem support and different forms of technical and informational support can help an athlete feel more confident in their ability to return to sport and address anxiety related concerns.

> *Straight after the operation I was stuck at home, couldn't really do anything, um, driving, couldn't drive anywhere, couldn't really do, do anything for myself, so it was, my life had to change significantly. Like where other people being like my parents and my brother helped me a lot more than they had done, you know I kind of went back to being like not a baby, but a toddler, that needed help with basic things like picking things up from the floor and stuff like that*
>
> *(Professional football player, cited in Arvinen-Barrow, 2009)*

Sources of social support

As suggested, the type of social support required may vary greatly, depending on various personal and situational factors surrounding individual athletes. Not only is it important to understand the types of support that might be beneficial and how these might meet an injured athlete's needs, it is also important to consider potential sources of social support (Figure 9.3).

During injury rehabilitation, athletes often associate and work with, a range of individuals who might act as sources of social support. These sources might be members of the athlete's immediate family, friends, sport team members (for example, coach, team mates) and sport medicine professionals (Heil, 1993b; Taylor

TABLE 9.1 Different types of social support during sport injury rehabilitation

Type of support	Description	References
Esteem	Enacting behaviours that bolster an athlete's self-confidence, sense of competence or self-esteem, perhaps through provision of positive feedback or by demonstrating belief in the athlete's ability to cope with injury	Freeman and Rees (2009) Rees (2007)
Listening	Actively listening to the athlete whilst refraining from giving advice or making judgement. This should involve sharing both positive (e.g. joys of rehabilitation success) and negative (e.g. setback frustrations) thoughts and feelings associated with rehabilitation	Taylor and Taylor (1997)
Emotional	Providing an athlete with impartial assistance during emotionally difficult times and demonstrating acceptance, empathy and encouragement should they experience setbacks, thus facilitating a sense of comfort and security	Freeman and Rees (2009) Rees, Mitchell, Evans, and Hardy (2010)
Emotional challenge	Challenging the athlete to do their utmost to overcome obstacles to goal-achievement, and structuring support so as to facilitate motivation toward rehabilitation	Taylor and Taylor (1997)
Shared social reality	Acting as a 'reality-touchstone' by verifying an athlete's perception of the current situation, and social context, thus potentially providing a sense of 'normalisation'	Taylor and Taylor (1997)
Technical appreciation	Demonstrating an acknowledgement of an athlete's achievements, or reinforcing effort and intensity during a rehabilitation session	Taylor and Taylor (1997)
Technical challenge	Encouraging athletes to achieve more, to be excited about their work and progress, and to seek new ways in which they might rehabilitate	Taylor and Taylor (1997)
Personal assistance	Providing advice, guidance, and assistance in the form of time, skill, knowledge and expertise targeted directly at problem-solving or feedback relating to rehabilitation	Rees et al. (2010)
Material assistance	Providing tangible assistance such as the provision of transport to rehabilitation, assistance with general household duties, and financial support thus directly facilitating an athlete's chances of goal achievement	Rees (2007) Rees et al. (2010)
Motivational	Encouraging athletes to overcome, or give into, various barriers during the rehabilitation process	Udry (2001, 2002)

and Taylor, 1997; Wagman and Khelifa, 1996). Depending on the role of each of these members during rehabilitation, together they will form the foundation for the primary and secondary rehabilitation teams working with the athlete during rehabilitation (for more details, see Chapter 11) in the hope of ensuring a fast return to pre-injury (or higher) levels of fitness and performance.

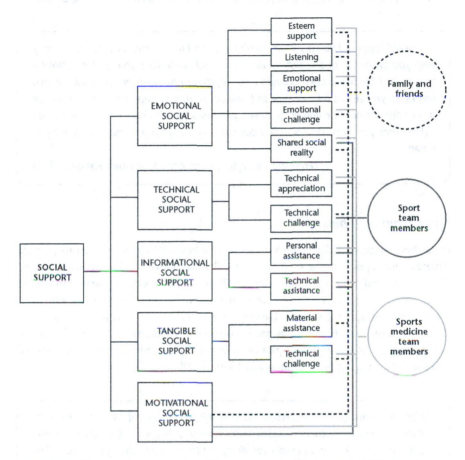

FIGURE 9.3 Types and sources of social support proposed as beneficial during the sport injury rehabilitation process

Source: collated from the works of Pines *et al.*, 1981; Udry, 1997, 2002

Family and friends

According to Taylor and Taylor (1997), family and friends are best suited to providing emotional and listening support, as well as support in the form of emotional challenge and shared social reality. Amongst professional rugby players, parents were also found to provide listening support, and emotional challenge support, to help players regain emotional control during difficult periods (Carson and Polman, 2008). Similarly, Arvinen-Barrow (2009) found that, amongst professional football and rugby players, families were seen as essential sources of emotional and motivational support. Moreover, when the injury resulted in major physical limitations, their role as a form of tangible support also increased (Arvinen-Barrow, 2009).

> *Um, well I suppose I had my family behind me, and my girlfriend as well, so... they help you an awful lot this um, cause it's a lonely time that you're in especially, I was in bed for two weeks I couldn't do anything just lying on my back for two weeks, so you've got a lot of time to think about things. Yeah I suppose, it can be a very depressing time and er, yeah you just need friends and family, it's essential, I think that you have that and without them you'd go mad, you'd go crazy you know*
>
> *(Professional rugby player, cited in Arvinen-Barrow, 2009)*

Sport team members

It has been suggested that team mates and coaches are best positioned to provide athletes with support in the form of technical appreciation, technical challenge and shared social reality (Taylor and Taylor, 1997). Research has demonstrated that team mates are also a source of inspiration (Carson and Polman, 2008) and a source of motivational support (Arvinen-Barrow, 2009). The coach's role has also been discussed in research literature, as professional coaches themselves view the provision of support as an important part of their role by providing emotional, material and informational support (Podlog and Eklund, 2007b).

> *I think that having another person, another injured player with you is quite vital. It makes it real to motivate yourself into training... because some days you feel like, I can't, I can't do it, I'm really too tired, but then your mate's, your mate's fine and he gets you through it."*
>
> *(A professional football player, cited in Arvinen-Barrow, 2009)*

Sport medicine team members

Much research suggests that sport medicine professionals may provide all types of social support, owing to their close relationship with athletes during injury rehabilitation (Taylor and Taylor, 1997). For example, Bianco (2001) found that sport medicine professionals were best suited to provide various types of emotional, informational and tangible support. A doctoral thesis by Arvinen-Barrow (2009) also found that, amongst professional rugby and association football players, those working with athletes on a daily basis were seen as important sources of emotional, informational and motivational support. Similarly, sport medicine professionals have been viewed as important sources of informational support, which enhances understanding of the injury and the rehabilitation process (Carson and Polman, 2008; Rock and Jones, 2002).

Researchers have also indicated that sport medicine professionals might facilitate athletes in seeking social support from additional sources, such as providing contacts to other injured athletes (see, for example, Arvinen-Barrow, Penny, Hemmings and Corr, 2010) or with allied health professionals. Other professional staff (typically classed as members of the secondary rehabilitation team; for more details, see Chapter 11) might also be important sources of social support. For example, Evans, Hardy and Flemming (2000) found that when setbacks occurred during rehabilitation, the use of a sport psychology consultant was particularly important.

Using social support for rehabilitation: the process

It appears that social support can influence reactions to the sport injury rehabilitation process directly and/or indirectly. It is also evident that there are different types of social support that are beneficial for injured athletes and that a number of individuals might represent useful sources of support. However, the extent to which each type of support is required and used by athletes can be dependent upon the support provider and the actual stage of rehabilitation (Bianco, 2001). It has also been suggested that having multiple sources of support available is important, as an athlete may then not feel limited to the potentially biased and/or unhelpful advice of one person (Carson and Polman, 2008).

There is currently little research that has examined how best to implement social support effectively within an injury context (Rees and Hardy, 2004) but it appears that social support might be provided in a number of ways (Freeman, Coffee and Rees, 2011). Mitchell (2011) and Rees (2007) have indicated that differing social support needs of injured athletes should be met through correspondingly different types of support, which should be provided at the right time and the right level for the process to be effective (Sarason *et al.*, 1990; Udry, 2001). This is supported by earlier suggestions from Richman, Hardy, Rosenfeld, and Callanan (1989), who proposed three general recommendations regarding the provision of support. According to the authors, social support:

1. is best provided by a network of individuals
2. needs to be developed and nurtured, and
3. works best as part of an ongoing programme rather than when employed purely as a reaction to a crisis.

Consequently, it has been suggested that support might be provided via peer modelling, which Kolt (2004) describes as the process of linking a currently injured athlete with another athlete who has undergone a similar rehabilitation process and who has recovered (or is nearly recovered) to their pre-injury performance level. Support for the use of peer modelling has been found in studies (for example, Wiese, Weiss and Yukelson, 1991) conducted with athletic trainers and injured athletes in the form of 'buddy systems' (Walker, 2006).

A further useful means of introducing social support is via injury support groups (Wiese *et al.*, 1991) or performance enhancement groups (Clement, Shannon and Connole, 2011). Often employed with athletes undergoing lengthy rehabilitation programmes, such groups can facilitate the establishment of important networks with other athletes and can offer opportunities to discuss experiences of injury and rehabilitation. Support groups have also been found to facilitate motivation (Weiss and Troxel, 1986), which can be a major factor in assisting athletes in reaching full recovery. Being part of a performance enhancement group can also teach athletes important psychological skills to help them cope with the distress caused by injury (Clement *et al.*, 2011). Given that social support as a concept, however, considers a range of social networks as potential sources of support, and that injured athletes have individual preferences for the sources of social support they consider benefi-cial, the use of peer modelling and injury support groups may not suit all. Thus, an alternative approach is one-to-one intervention (Freeman and Rees, 2009), which will often resemble a typical counselling relationship, whereby the effectiveness of the intervention is highly dependent on the nature of the working-alliance between the athlete and the support provider.

Social support: issues to consider

In addition to considering the potential types, sources, processes and mechanisms in which social support is best provided, we believe that those involved in social support provision should also consider:

- the characteristics of the support provider;
- the concept of perceived versus received support; and
- the negative effects of social support.

Characteristics of the support provider

Literature seems to suggest that individuals providing social support should possess certain intra- and interpersonal characteristics, skills and techniques in order for social support provision to be effective. Specifically, a person providing social support should: (1) be a good listener; (2) have the ability to identify personal and gender differences in athletes receiving support; (3) be able to acknowledge both effort and mastery; (4) with the help from systematic goal setting, be able to balance the use of technical appreciation and technical challenge; (5) possess awareness of social support as being the most necessary yet least available technique in relation to injury requiring surgery and lengthy rehabilitation; and (6) be able to identify correct intervention (such as support group or peer modelling) for individual athletes (see, for example, Heil, 1993a; Rees, 2007; Richman *et al.*, 1989; Taylor and Taylor, 1997; Udry, 2001).

The concept of perceived versus received support

In addition to the individual characteristics of the support provider, another consideration is the difference between perceived and received support. Bianco and Eklund (2001) highlighted that, for social support behaviours to occur, support networks must firstly be in place. Furthermore, the effectiveness of a support network is not necessarily associated with just the number of support providers available (Sarason *et al.*, 1990; Thoits, 1995) but, instead, is related to the extent to which various individuals recognise the need to provide support and are willing and able to provide support when necessary (Bianco and Eklund, 2001). Consequently, there are likely to be differences in the type of support that athletes require, expect to receive and actually receive, thus there will be variations depending upon the support provider and their role in the injured athlete's life, as well as the actual stage of rehabilitation (Bianco, 2001; Handegard, Joyner, Burke and Reimann, 2006). In addition, the timing of the support, injury type and injury severity can also impact upon an athlete's perception of required, provided and received social support (Taylor and Taylor, 1997). It has also been suggested that there might be gender differences in relation to the perceptions and use of social support; for example, female athletes have been perceived as having more emotional support available from their networks than male athletes (Hardy, Richman and Rosenfeld, 1991; Mitchell *et al.*, 2007; Rock and Jones, 2002).

Understanding the differences between perceived and actual support is important, as having a positive perception that support will be available when needed can influence appraisal of rehabilitation, as well as facilitate the development and use of effective coping skills. Increases in a supportive network, such as an increase in social integration, network size and frequency of contact with others in the network, are also associated with corresponding increases in positive outcomes (Rees, 2007). These positive outcomes might result from an athlete simply being part of a network, and as such their self-concept, self-worth and personal control might be enhanced.

Negative effects of social support

Although social support generally appears to have a positive influence, if provided insufficiently and inappropriately, it can have a negative effect on the athlete's overall health and wellbeing. Insufficient rehabilitation guidance, lack of sensitivity to the injury and lack of concern from those surrounding the athlete have been found to be negatively perceived by athletes (Udry, Gould, Bridges and Tuffey, 1997) and, as such, can be detrimental to the overall recovery process. Similarly, if the provider is not adequately skilled to provide the support needed or, indeed, is not aware of their role as a source of support, this could also have a negative effect on the athlete and the overall rehabilitation. Thus, those involved with athletes during injury rehabilitation should possess awareness of their possible role as a source of social support and also acknowledge their own competencies and limitations as potential providers of social support including an understanding of when to provide support and when not to.

Conclusion

Despite the lack of a distinct definition of social support, of all the psychological interventions available, social support appears to be one of the most used techniques during injury rehabilitation. Injured athletes appear to benefit from a range of different types of social support, provided by a number of individuals they typically associate with. This chapter has provided details of the mechanisms underlying the concept of social support, the different types and sources of social support that might be beneficial during rehabilitation and has discussed the range of potential sources of social support available during rehabilitation. Moreover, the chapter has outlined the process of using social support during rehabilitation and highlighted potential issues to consider when using social support with injured athletes.

CASE STUDY

John is a 35-year-old British international wheelchair tennis player. He lives with his wife, Emma, and their 24-month-old daughter, Elizabeth. Two and a half years ago, John was in a car accident and suffered a spinal cord injury and was later diagnosed with paraplegia. As a result, John has a total loss of movement and sensation in both legs. Before his accident, John was an amateur tennis player who just played for fun. After his accident, John has slowly come to terms with his lack of mobility and credits much of that to his tennis coach: 'if it wasn't for my coach helping me to discover wheelchair tennis, I am not sure where I would be now. I mean, after the accident I was in such a dark place. My wife was pregnant and I wasn't able to work, or provide, or even climb to bed without her help. What sort of a man was I, and what sort of a father would I be?'

Last week, John fell during a friendly match against his training partner and dislocated his right shoulder. Luckily, the team physiotherapist was at hand and John was able to receive appropriate first aid immediately. Following a doctor's consultation, it seems that John will not need surgery, provided that he is able to keep his arm resting and immobilised in a sling for at least a week. This should then be followed by mobility exercises and the use of the sling for at least another three to five weeks. The doctor also advised John that full return back to sport will take anywhere between 10 and 16 weeks, if he is able to ensure appropriate amounts of rest and immobilisation during the rehabilitation and recovery process.

John is obviously pleased about the possibility of avoiding surgery but also worried about his ability to cope with the injury appropriately. 'I mean, this is bad...how am I going to cope with all of this? Elizabeth is only small and I can't even pick her up now...or indeed wheel myself from one room to another! Why did my coach tell me to play this stupid friendly match anyway? It was so unnecessary and look where it got me!'

––––––––– **?** –––––––––

1. With reference to the integrated model of psychological response to sport injury and rehabilitation process (Wiese-Bjornstal *et al.*, 1998, see Chapter 3), highlight any key pre-injury factors and any possible personal and situational factors that can be seen as affecting John's appraisal of his injury?
2. Describe the types of social support that might be beneficial for John and explain why?
3. Describe who could be best suited to provide John with the different types of social support identified in question two to help facilitate his return to full fitness?

References

Arvinen-Barrow, M. (2009) Psychological rehabilitation from sport injury: Issues in the training and development of chartered physiotherapists. (Doctoral dissertation). University of Northampton. Retrieved from http://nectar.northampton.ac.uk/2456/

Arvinen-Barrow, M., Penny, G., Hemmings, B. and Corr, S. (2010) UK Chartered Physiotherapists' personal experiences in using psychological interventions with injured athletes: An interpretative phenomenological analysis. *Psychology of Sport and Exercise*, 11, 58–66.

Berkman, L. F. (1984) Assessing the physical health effects of social networks and social support. *Annual Review of Public Health*, 5, 413–32.

Bianco, T. (2001) Social support and recovery from sport injury: Elite skiers share their experiences. *Research Quarterly for Exercise and Sport*, 72, 376–88.

Bianco, T. and Eklund, R. (2001) Conceptual considerations for social support research in sport and exercise settings: The case of sport injury. *Journal of Sport and Exercise Psychology*, 23, 85–107.

Carson, F. and Polman, C. J. (2008) ACL injury rehabilitation: A psychological case study of a professional rugby union player. *Journal of Clinical Sport Psychology*, 2, 71–90.

Clement, D., Shannon, V. R. and Connole, I. J. (2011) Performance enhancement groups for injured athletes. *International Journal of Athletic Therapy & Training*, 16(3), 34–36.

Cohen, S. and Wills, T. A. (1985) Stress, social support, and the buffering hypothesis. *Psychological Bulletin*, 98, 310–357.

Cutrona, C. E. and Russell, D. W. (1990) Type of social support and specific stress: Toward a theory of optimal matching. In B. R. Sarason, I. G. Sarason and G. R. Pierce (eds), *Social Support: An interactional view*. New York: Wiley, pp. 319–36.

Evans, L., Hardy, L. and Flemming, S. (2000) Intervention strategies with injured athletes: An action research study. *The Sport Psychologist*, 14, 188–206.

Freeman, P. and Rees, T. (2009) How does perceived support lead to better performance? An examination of potential mechanisms. *Journal of Applied Sport Psychology*, 12(4), 429–41.

Freeman, P., Coffee, P. and Rees, T. (2011) The PASS-Q: The perceived available support in sport questionnaire. *Journal of Sport and Exercise Psychology*, 33, 54–74.

Fromm, E. (1955) *The Sane Society*. New York: Rinehart.

Gould, D., Finch, L. M. and Jackson, S. A. (1993) Coping strategies used by national champion figure skaters. *Research Quarterly for Exercise and Sport*, 64(4), 453–68.

Handegard, L. A., Joyner, A. B., Burke, K. L. and Reimann, B. (2006) Relaxation and guided imagery in the sport rehabilitation context. *Journal of Excellence*, 11, 146–64.

Hardy, C. J. and Grace, R. K. (1991) Social support within sport. *Sport Psychology Training Bulletin*, 3(1), 1–8.

Hardy, C. J. and Grace, R. K. (1993) The dimensions of social support when dealing with sport injuries. In D. Pargman (ed.), *Psychological Bases of Sport Injuries*. Morgantown, WV: Fitness Information Technology, pp. 121–44.

Hardy, C. J., Richman, J. M. and Rosenfeld, L. B. (1991) The role of social support in the life stress/injury relationship. *The Sport Psychologist*, 5, 128–39.

Hardy, L., Jones, G. and Gould, D. (1996) *Understanding Psychological Preparation for Sport: Theory and practice of elite performers*. Chichester: John Wiley & Sons.

Heil, J. (1993a) A comprehensive approach to injury management. In J. Heil (ed.), *Psychology of Sport Injury*. Champaign, IL: Human Kinetics, pp. 137–49.

Heil, J. (1993b) *Psychology of Sport Injury*. Champaign, IL: Human Kinetics.

Kolt, G. S. (2004) Injury from sport, exercise, and physical activity. In G. S. Kolt and M. B. Andersen (eds), *Psychology in the Physical and Manual Therapies*. London: Churchill Livingstone, pp. 247–67.

Litwak, E. and Szelenyi, I. (1969) Primary group structures and their functions: kin, neighbours and friends. *American Sociological Review*, 34, 465–81.

Maslow, A. H. (1954) *Motivation and Personality*. New York: Harper & Row.

Maslow, A. H. (1968) *Toward a Psychology of Being*. New York: Van Nostrand.

Mitchell, I. D. (2011) Social support and psychological responses in sport–injury rehabilitation. *Sport and Exercise Psychology Review*, 7(2), 30–44.

Mitchell, I. D., Neil, R., Wadey, R. and Hanton, S. (2007) Gender differences in athletes' social support during injury rehabilitation. *Journal of Sport & Exercise Psychology*, 29, S189–190.

Pines, A. M., Aronson, E. and Kafry, D. (1981) *Burnout*. New York: Free Press.

Podlog, L. and Eklund, R. C. (2007a) Professional coaches' perspectives on the return to sport following serious injury. *Journal of Applied Sport Psychology*, 19, 207–25.

Podlog, L. and Eklund, R. C. (2007b) Psychosocial considerations of the return to sport following injury. In D. Pargman (ed.), *Psychological Bases of Sport Injuries*, 3rd edn. Morgantown, WV: Fitness Information Technology, pp. 109–30.

Rees, T. (2007) Influence of social support on athletes. In S. Jowett and D. Lavallee (eds), *Social Psychology in Sport*. Champaign, IL: Human Kinetics, pp. 223–32.

Rees, T. and Freeman, P. (2007) The effects of perceived and received support on self-confidence. *Journal of Sports Sciences*, 25(9), 1057–65.

Rees, T. and Freeman, P. (2010) Social support and performance in a golf-putting experiment. *The Sport Psychologist*, 18, 333–48.

Rees, T. and Hardy, L. (2000) An investigation of the social support experiences of high-level sports performers. *The Sport Psychologist*, 14(4), 327–47.

Rees, T. and Hardy, L. (2004) Matching social support with stressors: Effects on factors underlying performance in tennis. *Psychology of Sport and Exercise*, 5, 319–37.

Rees, T., Hardy, L. and Freeman, P. (2007) Stressors, social support, and effects upon performance in golf. *Journal of Sports Sciences*, 25(1), 33–42.

Richman, J. M., Hardy, C. J., Rosenfeld, L. B. and Callanan, R. A. E. (1989) Strategies for enhancing social support networks in sport: A brainstorming experience. *Journal of Applied Sport Psychology*, 1, 150–59.

Rock, J. A. and Jones, M. V. (2002) A preliminary investigation into the use of counseling skills in support of rehabilitation from sport injury. *Journal of Sport Rehabilitation*, 11, 284–304.

Rotella, R. J. and Heyman, S. R. (1993) Stress, injury, and the psychological rehabilitation of athletes. In J. M. Williams (ed.), *Applied Sport Psychology: Personal growth to peak performance*, 2nd edn. Mountain View, CA: Mayfield, pp. 338–55.

Sarason, B. R., Sarason, I. G. and Gurung, R. A. R. (1997) Close personal relationships and health outcomes: A key to the role of social support. In S. Duck (ed.), *Handbook of Personal Relationships*. New York: Wiley, pp. 547–73.

Sarason, B. R., Sarason, I. G. and Pierce, G. R. (1990) Social support, personality, and performance. *Journal of Applied Sport Psychology*, 2, 117–27.

Taylor, J. and Taylor, S. (1997) *Psychological Approaches to Sports Injury Rehabilitation*. Gaithersburg, MD: Aspen.

Thoits, P. A. (1995) Stress, coping and social support processes: Where are we? What next? *Journal of Health and Social Behaviour*, Extra Issue, pp. 57–79.

Udry, E. (1997) Support providers and injured athletes: A specificity approach. *Journal of Applied Sport Psychology*, 9, S34.

Udry, E. (2001) The role of significant others: Social support during injuries. In J. Crossman (ed.), *Coping with Sports Injuries: Psychological strategies for rehabilitation*. Oxford: University Press, pp. 148–61.

Udry, E. (2002) Staying connected: Optimizing social support for injured athletes. *Athletic Therapy Today*, 7(3), 42–3.

Udry, E., Gould, D., Bridges, D. and Tuffey, S. (1997) People helping people? Examining the social ties of athletes coping with burnout and injury stress. *Journal of Sport and Exercise Psychology*, 19, 368–95.

Wagman, D. and Khelifa, M. (1996) Psychological issues in sport injury rehabilitation: Current knowledge and practice. *Journal of Athletic Training*, 31(3), 257–61.

Walker, N. (2006) *The Meaning of Sports Injury and Re-injury Anxiety Assessment and Intervention*. (Doctoral dissertation). University of Wales, Aberystwyth.

Weiss, M. R. and Troxel, R. K. (1986) Psychology of the injured athlete. *Athletic Training*, 21, 104–10.

Wiese, D. M., Weiss, M. R. and Yukelson, D. P. (1991) Sport psychology in the training room: A survey of athletic trainers. *The Sport Psychologist*, 5, 15–24.

Wiese-Bjornstal, D. M., Smith, A. M., Shaffer, S. M. and Morrey, M. A. (1998) An integrated model of response to sport injury: Psychological and sociological dynamics. *Journal of Applied Sport Psychology*, 10, 46–69.

PART 3

Delivering psychological interventions in sport injury rehabilitation

10

INTEGRATING THE PSYCHOLOGICAL AND PHYSIOLOGICAL ASPECTS OF SPORT INJURY REHABILITATION

Rehabilitation profiling and phases of rehabilitation

Cindra S. Kamphoff, Jeffrey Thomae and J. Jordan Hamson-Utley

Introduction

Over the last 20 years, the use of psychological interventions to speed recovery has become increasingly popular and vital in ensuring an athlete's a successful recovery and return to play (Ievleva and Orlick, 1991; Kamphoff *et al.*, 2010; Williams and Scherzer, 2010). The same psychological interventions that are used to help athletes to be successful in sports are being recommended to be implemented in the rehabilitation process (Williams and Scherzer, 2010). For non-injured athletes, psychological interventions like goal setting, positive self-talk, relaxation and imagery can be used consistently to enhance performance, increase enjoyment and achieve greater satisfaction in sport (Weinberg and Gould, 2007). Injured athletes may use psychological interventions for similar reasons, such as to increase enjoyment and satisfaction with the rehabilitation process, but they can also use psychological interventions to improve recovery time, facilitate physical recovery following surgery, buffer immune system deterioration, manage pain, prevent future injuries and improve adherence to rehabilitation (Ievleva and Orlick, 1991; Petrie and Hamson-Utley, 2011).

More specifically, researchers have found that athletes who used goal setting, imagery and positive self-talk recovered faster than athletes who did not use these psychological interventions in the rehabilitation process (Ievleva and Orlick, 1991). Other researchers have found that when injured athletes use psychological interventions, they experience a reduction in stress, pain, state anxiety and re-injury anxiety (Cupal, 1998; Loundagin and Fisher, 1993). Gould, Udry, Bridges and Beck (1997), for example, found that injured athletes who were able to return to pre-injury rankings thought that cognitive restructuring, positive self-talk and mental imagery were an essential part of their rehabilitation. Lastly, athletes who use these psychological interventions show a better adherence to rehabilitation (Evans and Hardy, 2002a; 2002b; for more details on different psychological interventions, see Chapters 5–9).

Sport medicine professionals and students have been taking note that being psychologically ready for competition may be as important as being physically ready to play (Hamson-Utley, Martin and Walters, 2008; Kamphoff *et al.*, 2010; Stiller-Ostrowski and Ostrowski, 2009). Yet, the majority of sport medicine professionals have tended not to incorporate psychological interventions into the rehabilitation programs of injured athletes (Arvinen-Barrow, Hemmings, Weigand, Becker and Booth, 2007; Clement, Granquist and Arvinen-Barrow, 2013; Larson, Starkey and Zaichkowsky, 1996; Washington-Lofren, Westerman, Sullivan and Nashman, 2004). Sport medicine professionals are in an important position to implement psychological interventions. Therefore, it is important for sport medicine professionals to be trained to understand and be able to use a wide array of psychology skills and interventions throughout the rehabilitation process (for example, Arvinen-Barrow, Hemmings, Becker and Booth, 2008).

To provide sport medicine professionals with the tools necessary to implement psychological interventions into the rehabilitation process, this chapter includes three distinct sections. Firstly, three phases of rehabilitation are outlined so that the sport medicine professional can create a plan of interventions based on typical physical and psychological aspects that pose challenges during each phase. Understanding these three phases allows sport medicine professionals to better assist the athlete and design psychological interventions specific for them to optimise recovery. Secondly, the concept of rehabilitation profiling (Taylor and Taylor, 1997) is outlined and how it can be used to better understand both the physical and psychological factors impacting the athlete and to effectively design interventions to buffer the negative effects of injury. It is recommended that rehabilitation profiling be implemented at several times during the rehabilitation process to better understand the athlete's perspective as well as the progress the athlete has made throughout rehabilitation. Lastly, and to support Part 2 of this book, five common psychological skills (goal setting, imagery, relaxation techniques, self-talk and social support) are discussed and specific recommendations are provided on when to introduce them into the different phases of rehabilitation.

> *I had worked so hard. I had left home when I was eleven for this sport. It's something that I love to do . . . I love it. I would think about not being able to play and break down completely; I would just be sobbing. I couldn't help myself, and I am not a crier . . . I took it really, really hard.*
>
> *(Nicholle's reaction to her injury, which demonstrates the importance of addressing rehabilitation from a holistic perspective [cited in Stoltenberg, Kamphoff and Lindstrom Bremer, 2010: 5])*

Three phases of rehabilitation: a holistic approach to healing the injured athlete

As demonstrated in Chapter 3, athletes will respond to injury in highly varied ways and it is helpful to consider a framework within which to facilitate an effective return to sport. When considering the rehabilitation process for the injured athlete, it is helpful to break it down into manageable phases, guided by distinct aspects of the healing process that may direct the use of specific psychological interventions to optimise recovery. There are three distinct phases: I) reaction to injury; II) reaction to rehabilitation; and III) reaction to return to play.

Phase I: reaction to injury

Phase I encapsulates the athlete's response to the injury, including physical and psychological factors (Hamson-Utley, 2010). Physically, the athlete will typically experience swelling, discoloration and pain resulting from tissue damage, which is dependent on the severity of injury. Also accompanying this stage is physical immobility, by which the athlete is forced to become inactive to a small or greater extent and may become dependent on others. Psychologically, during phase I, the athlete forms cognitive appraisals of the injury occurrence (positive or negative) and is consumed with the pain that the injury has produced. The athlete's lifestyle often changes to become more reliant on others, so less independent. As a result of the physical aspects of phase I, the athlete may experience anxiety and negative emotions surrounding the injury and be anxious about the recovery process. Highly useful psychological interventions in this phase include injury education and pain management which can be facilitated through goal setting, imagery and relaxation techniques.

Phase II: reaction to rehabilitation

When swelling, the range of motion (mobility) and levels of pain improve, this acts as a marker for the sport medicine professional that the athlete has progressed into phase II. This phase is characterised by the physical factors of strength, balance and mobility, and the psychological factors of motivation and hardiness (Hamson-Utley, 2010). Phase II of rehabilitation tends to be the most challenging for athletes as it is the longest phase for more severe injuries; an athlete with a ruptured ligament for example, may spend an average of three to four months in phase II. Psychologically, strategies that promote rehabilitation adherence and treatment compliance, motivate the athlete to work hard and highlight qualities of resilience in the athlete are best suited for this phase. Goal setting and self-talk would be the most relevant psychological interventions to use with the athlete to address these psychological concerns.

Phase III: reaction to return to play

The final phase of the rehabilitation process, phase III is marked physically by completing strength and proprioceptive (balance) gains and beginning sport-specific agility drills and movements (Hamson-Utley, 2010). Athletes may face additional physical roadblocks, such as the development of scar tissue in the injured joint, which causes a temporary setback in rehabilitation progress. How the sport medicine professional handles this is of upmost importance and is best managed through patient education and social support. Psychologically, in phase III the athlete deals primarily with self-confidence issues and managing their fears of re-injury as they approach their return to play. Useful psychological interventions for use during this phase include positive self-talk, performance imagery and goal setting.

Understanding the rehabilitation process through the athlete's eyes is important for those who are leading their injury recovery process to ensure an optimised approach. Methods should be both individualised and comprehensive to ensure that the athlete will heal at their body's physiological rate. The impact of roadblocks presented by physiological and psychological issues at each phase can be minimised through pairing the issue with an effective psychological intervention, thereby creating a holistic approach to injury rehabilitation.

Rehabilitation profiling

Performance profiling was introduced in the sport psychology literature in the early 1990s by Richard Butler and colleagues, as a way to better understand an athlete's perception of their ability and their preparation for performance (Butler, Smith and Irwin, 1993). The method includes two key concepts of applied sport psychology which are fundamental to performance: self-awareness and goal setting. Embedded in the framework of the personal construct theory (Kelly, 1963), the profiling system helps to determine the athlete's unique dimensions of their peak performance and their perception on these dimensions. Once the athlete completes the profiling, a goal setting process is followed.

The method has been applied to sport in various ways, including in the rehabilitation process (Taylor and Taylor, 1997). Within the rehabilitation process, Taylor and Taylor suggest assessing both the athlete's personal and physical factors that have an impact on both the time and quality of the rehabilitation process. Assessing both the personal and physical factors allows the sport medicine professional and athlete to gain a better sense of where the athlete rates him/herself on important factors that impact the rehabilitation process. The personal profile includes 12 psychological, emotional and social factors including confidence, motivation, anxiety, focus, expectations, worry, emotions, identity, adherence, understanding, pain tolerance and social support (Figure 10.1 and Table 10.1).

The physical profile includes 12 injury-specific and health-related factors, including range of motion, strength, stability, coordination, balance, swelling, pain,

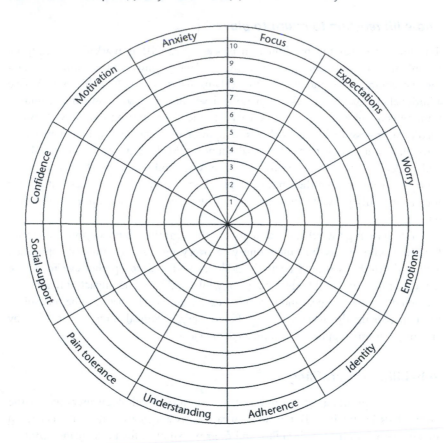

FIGURE 10.1 Rehabilitation profiling: personal profile

Source: adapted from Taylor and Taylor, 1997

function, daily activities, sports participation, health and sleep (Figure 10.2 and Table 10.2).

To begin the assessment, the factor descriptions should be read and understood by both the athlete and the sport medicine professional (see Tables 10.1 and 10.2). The athlete assesses their current perceptions, shading from the middle toward the outside of each of the 12 scales (see Figure 10.3 for an example).

There are many benefits of using the profile system when working with an athlete through the rehabilitation process. By taking into account the athlete's strengths and weakness, the sport medicine professional can tailor a unique set of interventions to the individual according to the current phase of rehabilitation and positively impact the athlete's adherence to the rehabilitation program. Additional benefits of such a process include:

TABLE 10.1 Rehabilitation profiling: definition of personal factors

Personal factor	Description	Score
Confidence	The degree of how much you believe in your ability during rehabilitation	0 = very low 10 = very high
Motivation	Your current level of motivation in your rehabilitation	0 = very low 10 = very high
Anxiety	The degree of physical anxiety you experience about your recovery	0 = considerable 10 = none
Focus	The degree to which you stay focused on your rehabilitation	0 = negative or distracted 10 = positive or focused
Expectations	The degree of positive expectations you have about your recovery	0 = low 10 = high
Worry	The degree of uneasiness, concern, and doubt you have about your recovery	0 = considerable 10 = none
Emotions	The degree you feel emotional about your rehabilitation	0 = very low or negative 10 = very high or positive
Identity	The degree you currently view yourself as a physical being and athlete	0 = very negatively 10 = very positively
Adherence	The degree to which you adhere to your rehabilitation programme	0 = very negatively 10 = very positively
Understanding	The degree of understanding you have of the rehabilitation process	0 = none 10 = considerable
Pain tolerance	The degree to which you can tolerate and control pain during rehabilitation	0 = very poorly 10 = very well
Social support	The degree of social support you are receiving from others including the sport medicine professionals, family, friends, coaches and team mates	0 = none 10 = considerable

Source: adapted from Taylor and Taylor, 1997

- The rehabilitation profiling system allows the sport medicine professional and athlete to better understand their psychological and physical needs of the athlete.
- Once completed, the athlete has a graphic representation of where they are in the rehabilitation process, both physically and psychologically, and it can then be used to determine the athlete's needs and goals.
- The athlete will increase their knowledge of the physical and psychological factors impacting the rehabilitation process which could impact their self-determination or their belief that they have control over their own actions and destiny.
- The profiling system provides an understanding of which psychological issues will both help and hinder the rehabilitation process.

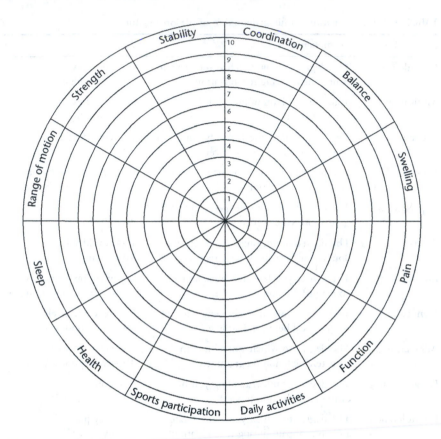

FIGURE 10.2 Rehabilitation profiling: physical profile

Source: adapted from Taylor and Taylor, 1997

- Over time, a series of profiles can demonstrate goal achievement to the athlete and can help with persistence throughout rehabilitation and in the return to competition.
- The profiling system is based on the athlete's perception of factors that are impacting the rehabilitation process. This provides a window into the lived experience of the injured athlete and, at the same time, provides an inroad for further development of the helping relationship. This insight can also provide important clues to potential barriers to the rehabilitation process.
- If an assessment such as the profiling system is not used, the sport medicine professional may miss important information that impacts the athlete and their engagement in rehabilitation.
- It is suggested that the sport medicine professional will be more effective in working with the athlete if an assessment like the rehabilitation profiling system is used.

TABLE 10.2 Rehabilitation profiling: definition of physical factors

Physical factor	Description	Score
Range of motion	The degree of quantity and quality of movement that you have in the injured area of the proximal or distal joint	0 = 0%, 10 = 100%
Strength	The degree or amount of force you can generate through the injured area	0 = 0%, 10 = 100%
Stability	The degree of firmness and steadiness you feel in the injured area	0 = 0%, 10 = 100%
Coordination	The degree to which you use different muscle groups together to produce a certain movement	0 = none; 10 = completely
Balance	The degree to which you can maintain equilibrium that is required to the injured area	0 = none; 10 = completely
Swelling	The degree of amount of fluid you have in the injured area	0 = considerable, 10 = none
Pain	The degree of discomfort and soreness that you feel in the injured area	0 = considerable, 10 = none
Function	The degree to which you can carry out sport-related activities involving the injured area	0 = not at all; 10 = completely
Daily activities	The degree to which you can carry out typical daily activities	0 = not at all; 10 = completely
Sports participation	The degree to which you can participate in your normal sport activities	0 = none; 10 = completely
Health	The degree of general good health you have, free of fatigue, illness, or minor injuries	0 = poor; 10 = excellent
Sleep	The degree of how much you are sleeping	0 = very poorly; 10 = very well

Source: adapted from Taylor and Taylor, 1997

Reasons to use rehabilitation profiling

1. The sport medicine professional will be able to better design a more effective rehabilitation programme for the athlete.
2. The sport medicine professional will have a better understanding of the psychological and physical needs of the athlete.
3. The athlete will have a graphic representation of where they are in the rehabilitation process both physically and psychologically.
4. The sport medicine professional will be able to determine the athlete's needs and goals.

5. The sport medicine professional will have a better understanding of which psychological issues will both help and hinder the rehabilitation process.
6. If an assessment is not used, the sport medicine professional may miss important information that impacts the athlete and their engagement in rehabilitation.
7. In general, the sport medicine professional will be more effective in working with the athlete.

(Gould, 1993)

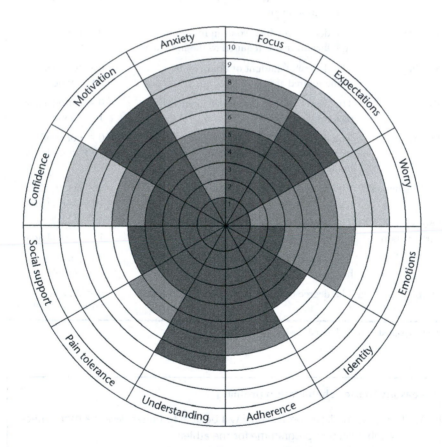

Key: dark grey = phase 1, middle grey = phase 2, light grey = phase 3

FIGURE 10.3 An example of changes in the rehabilitation profile across the three phases of rehabilitation

Source: adapted from Taylor and Taylor, 1997

Once the athlete has completed the two profiles, it is suggested that the sport medicine professional and the athlete discuss the athlete's ratings on each of the factors, beginning with those rated highest. This allows the athlete to explore their strengths and may provide an opportunity for additional development of the relationship between the sport medicine professional and the athlete. Then, the sport medicine professional should discuss the factors which the athlete rated lower. Once that discussion has taken place, together the athlete and sport medicine professional should determine where the athlete would like to improve within a specified timeframe. The sport medicine professional and athlete could use the form available as Figure 10.4 to set goals, after determining and discussing the athlete's strengths and weaknesses (for an overview of the goal setting process, see Chapter 5).

Furthermore, the rehabilitation profiling system has an advantage of providing a means of having one format for the athlete and sport medicine professional to periodically assess and record the athlete's progress. We suggest that the first rehabilitation profile should be completed by the athlete at least 72 hours following the injury occurrence. This allows the athlete to gain perspective regarding the injury and to attend to immediate physical and psychological needs, so as to be able to attend to learning a new psychological skill as a coping mechanism for healing. It would be appropriate for the athlete to complete the rehabilitation profiling system again between phases I and II as well as between phases II and III (see section below describing the three stages of the rehabilitation process). Additionally, depending on how long the athlete's phase II lasts, the athlete could take the assessment multiple times throughout the phase. The sport medicine professional should look for changes in the athlete's behaviour and use this as a guide for distributing the profile again.

It is suggested that the first rehabilitation profile should be completed by the athlete at least 72 hours following the injury occurrence.

By continuing to use the rehabilitation profile throughout the rehabilitation process, it provides a means of monitoring change. The athlete will also see the changes they have made throughout the stages of rehabilitation, potentially building their self-efficacy. By repeating the rehabilitation profiling system, the sport medicine professional and athlete will also be able to see visually which goals have been met. The hope is that, throughout the rehabilitation process, the athlete would cover more of the circle or profile. Figure 10.3, for instance, provides an example of an athlete who has made several perceived changes in her personal profile throughout her three phases of rehabilitation, including a higher confidence, focus, positive expectations, positive emotions, adherence and pain tolerance. The athlete has also experienced less anxiety and worry towards the end of her rehabilitation (note that anxiety and worry is reversed scored on the profile so that more covered on the profile indicates less of both concepts). Many of the variables remained

Directions: In the space below, indicate up to five factors from the personal profile on which you want to focus in your psychological rehabilitation. Then specify several strategies you will use to improve these areas and the timeframe in which you would like to improve.

Personal profile area identified	Strategies for improvement	Timeframe of goal

FIGURE 10.4 Rehabilitation goal sheet

Source: adapted from Taylor and Taylor, 1997

consistent in this athlete's rehabilitation including motivation, social support, understanding and identity.

We would expect that many important changes would occur in both the personal and physical profiles of which it is important to take note as a sport medicine professional. Meaning, all of the physical factors should improve throughout the three phases, such as the athlete's range of motion, strength, stability, coordination and balancing. Similarly, it is also expected that the athlete's confidence would increase throughout the three phases of rehabilitation, whereas their worry may or may not be steady. Based on research, the sport medicine professional may also expect some gender and cultural differences when working with athletes during the rehabilitation process. Clement *et al.* (2012), for example, found that male athletes with no past experience working with a sport medicine professional had lower expectations of personal commitment to the rehabilitation process and did expect sport medicine professionals to provide a facilitative environment. Furthermore, female athletes with experience of working with a sport medicine professional were least likely to have realistic expectations of sport medicine and injury rehabilitation. In addition, Clement *et al.* (2013) found a significant difference in mental skills usage during rehabilitation by country. That is, a greater proportion of athletes from the United States (33.4%) reported that they used mental skills during rehabilitation compared with athletes from the United Kingdom (23.4%) and Finland (20.3%).

Incorporating psychological skills into the three phases of rehabilitation

As has been established throughout this chapter, individual interventions should be tailored to the specific phase of rehabilitation for injured athletes and which reflect their unique personal and physical profiles. The following brief discussion of five common psychological interventions, in combination with later chapters in this text, provides the sport medicine professional with tools to match the psychological intervention to the needs of the athlete within each phase.

Incorporating goal setting into the three phases of rehabilitation

As demonstrated in Chapter 5, goal setting can play an important role in the injury rehabilitation process. Goal setting as a psychological intervention can be used throughout the three phases of rehabilitation. Understanding the types of goals, their relationship to an increased sense of control and self-determination and educating athletes on how to construct effective goals are all relevant concepts throughout the three phases of rehabilitation.

Phase I

As discussed above, injury education and the management of pain are critical psychological aspects of this phase. Thus, goal setting in this phase is likely to be broad in scope (for example, surgery to repair a torn labrum is likely to last three to four months and should allow for some sport-related exercise after about six weeks) as sport medicine professionals work with the athlete to understand the injury as well as the process of rehabilitation and the return the sport. Athletes must be told (and reminded) that their success in meeting goals for these broad recovery outcomes is contingent upon their effort and engagement in the rehabilitation process on a daily basis. Regarding the management of pain, athletes could use either association or disassociation techniques to manage their pain. Exercises can be as simple as diverting their attention to an informational video on an iPad or to the ESPN broadcast on the television wall while completing a painful range of motion exercise (disassociation) or teaching the athlete to gain control over their pain by imaging their pain as the volume on a stereo on which they can turn down the dial when pain is too much to handle (association). Either way, teaching the athlete pain coping skills during phase I will likely come in handy in future phases.

Phase II

Generally the longest phase of rehabilitation, phase II is when athletes will benefit significantly from goal setting. Using the principles of successful goals (see Chapter 5) can help to create a positive motivational climate in which athletes engage more fully in the rehabilitation process and adhere to a rehab program. Goal setting in this phase allows athletes to have measurable evidence of their progress and should be flexible enough to encourage adherence even in the face of setbacks. It is important to involve athletes in the goal setting process throughout this phase, to increase their sense of autonomy and self-determination over the process. Motivation is of utmost importance in this phase of rehabilitation and setting accurate goals will assist in motivating the athlete to continue therapy.

Phase III

One of the benefits of successful goal setting in phases I and II is that it can serve as evidence of the athlete's effort and success in rehabilitation to leverage into their return to sport. Goal setting in this phase can also be used during the transition back to practice or competition so that athletes do not apply an inappropriate amount of stress too early in their return. It can provide them with a period to build confidence as they test their injury.

Incorporating imagery into the three phases of rehabilitation

As Chapter 6 demonstrates, imagery is an important tool injured athletes can use in their injury rehabilitation, particularly because it can be done when time spent 'on the court' is limited by injury. Imagery can be used in any of the three phases of injury rehabilitation, shifting focus with each phase.

Phase I

In the initial wake of an injury, pain management and dealing with the loss of function is particularly salient to athletes. Imagery interventions during this phase should focus on two major areas: pain management and healing. There are a number of ways in which imagery can be used to assist in the management of pain. Imagery for pain management should emphasise vivid, polysensory images that can help athletes to exhibit control over the perception of the pain they are feeling. Imagery scripts in this phase might emphasise the reduction of swelling (imagining superabsorbent materials drawing fluid away from the injured area), muscle repair (imagining muscle fibres knitting back together, weaving strong and resilient new fibres into the healing muscles) or mending bones (imagining the bone healing with super-strong carbon fibre materials). Additionally, imagery exercises can help athletes 'dial down' a hot colour or loud sound associated with the pain they are feeling, shifting to cooler colours or quieter sounds associated with less pain (Hamson-Utley, 2012). Similarly, imagining the ability to expel pain with each breath the athlete exhales can provide another image for pain management.

Phase II

During the main rehabilitation phase of the injury, the athlete has regained much of the function from the injury but continues to engage in sometimes gruelling rehabilitation exercises and interventions. In addition to continuing healing imagery during this phase, one can also shift to imagery focused on success in rehabilitation sessions. For example, an athlete could use imagery the night before or the day of rehab to rehearse success in completing individual rehabilitation exercises with proper form. Similar to healing imagery mentioned above, athletes can spend time focusing on how rehabilitation sessions are continuing to strengthen the injured area and building the confidence for phase III, the return to sport.

Phase III

In preparing for a return to their sport, imagery should focus on the sensations associated with successfully performing skills at the level they did prior to the injury. In a sport like basketball, for example, with many sharp direction changes in response to opponents' movements, rich images of success in those actions can alleviate the anxiety many athletes have about re-injury and can build confidence. Performance imagery that recalls successful sport images is often used in this phase to build confidence in the athlete that they are ready to take the field. The athlete can also benefit from positive self-talk and pre-practice or pre-game imagery routines.

Incorporating relaxation techniques into the three phases of rehabilitation

The ability to produce physical relaxation throughout the body and specifically in the injured area is a foundational skill to other psychological interventions discussed throughout this text (for more details on relaxation techniques, see Chapter 7). Relaxation is a must for imagery interventions, for example, because it reduces both cognitive and somatic anxiety, allowing the athlete to focus fully on rehabilitation (Flint, 1998). Athletes may have little or no experience with physical relaxation as a skill when they first become injured and start the rehabilitation process. Sport medicine professionals delivering rehabilitation services to injured athletes should, therefore, become skilled in helping athletes gain competence in physical relaxation.

Phase I

Physical relaxation is an important initial intervention immediately after athletic injury because muscle tension contributes to increased experience of pain. This experience of pain, and efforts to manage it, can be consuming to an athlete and efforts to develop relaxation skills should focus on pain management during phase I. Physical relaxation interventions are predicated on having calm, quiet, inviting spaces in which to learn and practice and pose a challenge to professionals whose rehabilitation facilities have significant traffic and noise (Walsh, 2011). Carving out spaces away from the hustle and bustle within rehabilitation facilities is critical to the success of a relaxation intervention. In this phase, sport medicine professionals can teach athletes deep-breathing techniques and the repetition of words, phrases, sounds or prayers to induce a state of relaxation (Walsh, 2011).

Phase II

While relaxation interventions during phase I focus on pain management, interventions during Phase II should focus on the stress response to injury. Building on the skills developed in phase I, athletes are more efficient in inducing relaxation in the body, which can help to manage cognitive anxiety associated with the uncertainty of knowing when they will be able to return to competition or if they will make it back at all (Walsh, 2011). In phase II, athletes can use physical relaxation techniques in tandem with imagery to increase effort and persistence, as well as manage soreness and pain associated with the long hours of rehabilitation exercises.

Phase III

As athletes look forward to returning to competition in their sport, anxiety and stress responses can increase. As discussed above, the ability to induce a state of physical relaxation is an important skill and should be emphasised in response to the normal increase of anxiety during this phase. Once physical relaxation is mastered, more emphasis can be directed toward imagery and self-talk.

Incorporating positive self-talk into the three phases of rehabilitation

The quality of an injured athlete's cognitions before, during and after injury, including rehabilitation and return to sport, has been shown to be a critical piece of the psychological response to injury (see Chapter 3 for a discussion of relevant models). An athlete's self-talk is likely to change a great deal throughout the process and interventions can be targeted accordingly (see Chapter 8 for more details).

Phase I

In the immediate aftermath of an injury, an athlete is likely to experience a variety of normal but unhelpful negative thoughts about the significance of his or her injury ('My knee is gone.'), the significance of the injury to future success ('My career is over.') and may blame others ('Coach made me do that vault even thought I didn't want to.') (Flint, 1998). In addition, the athlete may be struggling to cope with the pain of the injury and the prospect of a difficult rehabilitation process. Self-talk interventions in this early stage should focus on the ability to manage pain successfully, and should begin to focus on an optimistic approach and adherence to rehabilitation. Affirmations can be helpful self-talk strategies ('I'm strong' or 'I can handle this'). In addition, distraction can help direct thoughts away from the experience of pain, lessening its impact.

Phase II

Throughout the bulk of rehabilitation, self-talk should focus on motivation to persist in the face of difficult rehabilitation exercises. While the general progress of rehabilitation is positive, that process will not be without its good days and bad days and can challenge athletes to remain positive. Focusing on self-talk that reinforces effort, persistence and success is critical. An athlete might focus on thoughts like 'I'm choosing to rehab today, and will try my hardest at each rep!'.

Phase III

Self-talk interventions can help athletes to manage anxiety and doubt about their return to competition. In particular, self-talk can focus athletes on thoughts associated with successfully performing the skills they need. Similarly, building a self-affirming self-talk that builds confidence for the return is critical. Focusing on thoughts like 'I worked hard at rehabilitation', 'My knee is strong', 'I'm excited to come back and show my team mates I'm ready!' can reduce doubt and uncertainty that is often experienced as athletes face the return to sport.

Incorporating social support into the three phases of rehabilitation

Social support has been shown to have a significant role in both predicting injury (Williams and Andersen, 2007) and the psychological response to injury (Wiese-Bjornstal, Smith, Shaffer and Morrey, 1998). Throughout the phases of rehabilitation, strong support from an athlete's family, friends, team mates, coaches and/or sport medicine professionals can facilitate positive rehab outcomes by reducing stress and increasing motivation (for more details, see Chapter 9).

Phase I

Injury challenges athletes in many ways, not the least of which is the potential loss of their athletic identity, owing to an inability to compete in their sport. In addition, athletes facing first-time and/or serious injury may struggle to understand the injury itself, as well as the process of rehabilitation and return to sport. Depending on the location and severity of an injury, athletes may struggle to meet the demands of day-to-day living because of mobility concerns. All of this can cause significant stress to an injured athlete. Helping him or her identify meaningful sources of support becomes a focus during this phase.

After injury, college athletes reported an increase in perceived social support from athletic trainers, coaches and physicians (Yang, Peek-Asa, Lowe, Heiden and Foster, 2010). While this finding is unsurprising, given the increased time spent with those professionals, it underscores the importance of attending to an athlete's social support needs throughout the process and particularly during the initial stages of injury rehabilitation. Sport medicine professionals delivering rehab services need to take time early on to ensure that athletes have identified sources of support and provide informational support if athletes' support needs are not being met.

Phase II

Throughout the lengthy middle phase athletes' rehabilitation process, healing continues, athletes gain use of the injured area and thus early concerns about day-to-day functioning lessen. Sources of social support during this phase should focus on helping athletes to cope with the daily challenges of being successful in meeting rehabilitation goals and dealing with normal setbacks throughout the process. Of particular concern to many team-sport athletes is the continued connection to team mates and the redefinition of their role on the team. Team captains who become injured, for example, may find their leadership role shifting to others and may struggle with less contact and the feeling of not being 'in the trenches' with team mates. Rehabilitation professionals should be aware of the potential for injury and rehabilitation to contribute to an athlete's sense of estrangement. Collaborating with coaches to help injured athletes continue to contribute in meaningful ways to the team can help maintain the social cohesion with team mates and, in turn, maintain critical sources of social support.

Phase III

As rehabilitation progresses to the point where strength and agility are dominant physical concerns, athletes may continue to experience the ups and downs of rehabilitation. With the return to sport close at hand, doubts about readiness and self-confidence about competitive success require sport medicine professionals to take the role of encouragers and confidence-builders. When doubt appears, sport medicine professionals can redirect athletes to focus on the effort they have put into their rehabilitation and the success they have had in that process. Research has shown that when sport medicine professionals provide a productive optimism and listen closely to the athlete this can be helpful (Naylor, 2007). For example, a sport medicine professional in this phase who sighs and avoids eye contact when she/he says, 'Well, we'll see how it goes' communicates a great deal to the athlete that can affect the way that athlete perceives the support of the sport medicine professional. On the other hand, the athlete would likely rate the sport medicine professional's support differently if she/he says, 'The ups and downs you are experiencing are normal and if you continue to put the effort I've seen so far, I'm confident you'll make it back physically and psychologically stronger than you were before your injury'.

Implications for sport medicine professionals: the conclusion

The responsibility of the professionals treating the athletes during rehabilitation is to support the athlete to return to play in the best possible way. To do this, the athlete must be both physically and mentally ready and the professionals responsible for the rehabilitation should have a role in ensuring this takes place. In fact, the current trend in sport-injury rehabilitation suggests focusing on a holistic approach, in which the sport medicine professional must integrate the physical and psychological skills in the three phases of rehabilitation (Hamson-Utley, 2010).

This chapter has provided direction for the sport medicine professional so they can better understand the athlete's perception and factors that would impact their rehabilitation, by describing the three phases of rehabilitation. In addition, by using rehabilitation profiling, the sport medicine professional can better understand the athlete's perception of both personal and physical factors that impact on the rehabilitation process and to ensure an optimised approach. Once the profile is complete, a discussion can take place and together, the athlete and sport medicine professional can determine where the athlete would like to improve within a specified timeframe.

Rehabilitation profiling can also be used throughout the three phases of rehabilitation to track the athlete's progress and set new goals. Using rehabilitation profiling, the psychological interventions could be chosen to ensure the athlete receives the most out of the rehabilitation process. Psychological interventions should also be introduced to create a holistic approach to injury rehabilitation which will increase adherence, improve their positive outlook, reduce pain, increase satisfaction, improve relaxation and decrease recovery time (Driediger, Hall and Callow, 2006; Evans, Hare and Mullen, 2006; Monsma, Mensch and Farroll, 2009; Rotella, Hedgpeth and Pickens, 1999).

The sport medicine professional can provide a key role in introducing the five common psychological interventions (goal setting, imagery, relaxation techniques, self-talk, and social support) discussed in this chapter to address these benefits. As more and more athletes use psychological interventions regularly in their season, they bring prior experience with psychological interventions to incorporate in the rehabilitation process (Hamson-Utley, 2010). This prior experience makes it more straightforward for the sport medicine professional to address both the physical and mental components to fully rehabilitation the injured athlete.

Using psychological interventions in the three phases of rehabilitation

Phase I: Reaction to injury. Physical relaxation is an important initial intervention immediately after athletic injury because muscle tension contributes to increased experience of pain. Similarly, healing imagery is a particularly potent psychological intervention in the initial stages as athletes deal with the pain and swelling associated with injury. Goal setting can assist athletes gain perspective and focus on a plan for recovery.

Phase II: Reaction to rehabilitation. Measuring progress toward goals set initially is critical for maintaining motivation during rehabilitation. Confronting negative or irrational thoughts and replacing them with affirming and positive thoughts is also an important part of this phase. Sport medicine professionals can also provide social support during this phase to help athletes to cope with the daily challenges of meeting rehabilitation goals and dealing with normal setbacks throughout the process.

Phase III: Reaction to return to play. The use of imagery and self-talk to build confidence can help an athlete be as mentally ready to return to sport as rehabilitation has helped prepare their body. During this stage, it is also important that the sport medicine professional takes on a role of encourager and confidence-builder by providing social support and reassurance.

CASE STUDY

Kerri is a talented ice hockey goalkeeper starting her fourth and last year of collegiate eligibility. After a history of problems with shoulder dislocations, she opted to have surgery to repair her labrum during the summer. The surgery was successful and doctors seemed confident that Kerri would be able to return to hockey-related exercises within about six weeks and fully healed within three to four months. The only complicating factor in this early stage was the intensity of the post-surgical pain she experienced, which she struggled to manage. She said that she often dreams about hockey, often with images of watching opponents making shots on goal while she can't move her arms to stop them.

In early rehabilitation sessions, Kerry talked at length with the sport medicine staff that she was driven to return quickly. In fact, the sport medicine professional working with her has had to talk to her about not pushing too hard too early in her rehab. She mentioned that she's thinking about rehabilitation all the time and is anxious about making a full recovery. She reports struggling with sleep because she's worried that losing the starting position as the team's goalkeeper would mean that she'll lose an opportunity to be scouted for the upcoming Olympic team.

1. How would you use the rehabilitation profiling as a sport medicine professional when working with Kerri?
2. What would you expect that Kerri would experience as she progresses through the three stages of rehabilitation? Why?
3. Which psychological skills would be important for you to introduce to Kerri as she progresses through the three stages of rehabilitation? Why? How would you introduce these psychological skills?

References

Arvinen-Barrow, M., Hemmings, B., Becker, C. A. and Booth, L. (2008) Sport psychology education: A preliminary survey into chartered physiotherapists' preferred methods of training delivery. *Journal of Sport Rehabilitation*, 17(4), 399–412.

Arvinen-Barrow, M., Hemmings, B., Weigand, D. A., Becker, C. A. and Booth, L. (2007) Views of chartered physiotherapists on the psychological content of their practice: A national follow-up survey in the United Kingdom. *Journal of Sport Rehabilitation*, 16, 111–21.

Butler, R. J., Smith, M. and Irwin, I. (1993) The performance profile in practice. *Journal of Applied Sport Psychology*, 5, 48–63.

Clement, D., Granquist, M. and Arvinen-Barrow, M. (2013) Psychosocial aspects of athletic injuries as perceived by athletic trainers. *Journal of Athletic Training*.

Clement, D., Hamson-Utley, J. J., Arvinen–Barrow, M., Kamphoff, C., Zakrajsek, R. A. and Martin, S. B. (2012) College athletes' expectations about injury rehabilitation with an athletic trainer. *International Journal of Athletic Therapy & Training*, 17(4), 18–27.

Cupal, D. D. (1998) Psychological interventions in sport injury prevention and rehabilitation. *Journal of Applied Sport Psychology*, 10(1), 103–23.

Driediger, M., Hall, C. and Callow, N. (2006) Imagery use by injured athletes: A qualitative analysis. *Journal of Sports Sciences*, 24(3), 261–71.

Evans, L. and Hardy, L. (2002a) Injury rehabilitation: A goal setting intervention study. *Research Quarterly for Exercise and Sport*, 73, 310–19.

Evans, L. and Hardy, L. (2002b) Injury rehabilitation: A qualitative follow-up study. *Research Quarterly for Exercise and Sport*, 73, 320–9.

Evans, L., Hare, R. and Mullen, R. (2006) Imagery use during rehabilitation from injury. *Journal of Imagery Research in Sport and Physical Activity*, 1(1), Article 1. doi:10.2202/1932-0191.1000

Flint, F. (1998) *Psychology of Sport Injury: A professional achievement self-study program course.* Champaign, IL: Human Kinetics.

Gould, D. (1993) Goal setting for peak performance. In J. Williams (ed.), *Applied Sport Psychology: Personal growth to peak performance.* Palo Alto, CA: Mayfield, pp. 158–69.

Gould, D., Udry, E., Bridges, D. and Beck, L. (1997) Coping with season-ending injuries. *The Sport Psychologist*, 11, 379–99.

Hamson-Utley, J. J. (2010) Psychology of sport injury: A holistic approach to rehabilitating the injured athlete. *Chinese Journal of Sports Medicine*, 29(3), 343–7.

Hamson-Utley, J. J. (2012) Athletic training – Dr. Jordan Hamson-Utley. [Audio podcast]. Retrieved from http://itunes.apple.com/us/podcast/athletic-training-dr.-jordan/id337761098

Hamson-Utley, J. J., Martin, S. and Walters, J. (2008) Athletic trainers' and physical therapists' perceptions of the effectiveness of psychological skills within sport injury rehabilitation programs. *Journal of Athletic Training*, 43(3), 258–64.

Ievleva, L. and Orlick, T. (1991) Mental links to enhanced healing: An exploratory study. *The Sport Psychologist*, 5, 25–40.

Kamphoff, C., Hamson-Utley, J. J., Antoine, B., Knutson, B., Thomae, J. and Hoenig, C. (2010) Athletic training students' perceptions of the importance and effectiveness of psychological skills within sport injury rehabilitation. *Athletic Training Education Journal*, 5(3), 109–16.

Kelly, G. A. (1963) *A Theory of Personality.* New York: W. W. Norton.

Larson, G. A., Starkey, C. and Zaichkowsky, L. D. (1996) Psychological aspects of athletic injuries as perceived by athletic trainers. *The Sport Psychologist*, 10, 37–47.

Loundagin, C. and Fisher, L. (1993) *The relationship between mental skills and enhanced athletic injury rehabilitation.* Paper presented at the Annual Meeting of the Association for the Advancement of Applied Sport Psychology and the Canadian Society for Psychomotor Learning and Sport Psychology, Montreal, Canada.

Monsma, E., Mensch, J. and Farroll, J. (2009) Keeping your head in the game: Sport-specific imagery and anxiety among injured athletes. *Journal of Athletic Training*, 44(4), 410–7.

Naylor, A. H. (2007) The Key to Committed Rehabilitation. *Athletic Therapy Today*, 12(3), 14.

Petrie, T. A. and Hamson-Utley, J. J. (2011) Psychosocial antecedents of and responses to athletic injury In T. Morris and P. Terry (eds), *Sport and Exercise Psychology: The cutting edge.* Morgantown, WV: Fitness Information Technology, pp. 531–51.

Rotella, R., Hedgpeth, E. G. and Pickens, M. (1999) The psychology of injury and rehabilitation. In D. H. Perrin (ed.), *The Injured Athlete.* Philadelphia, PA: Lippincott-Raven, pp. 175–86.

Stiller-Ostrowski, J. L. and Ostrowski, J. A. (2009) Recently certified athletic trainers' undergraduate educational preparation in psychosocial intervention and referral. *Journal of Athletic Training*, 44, 67–75.

Stoltenberg, A., Kamphoff, C. and Lindstrom Bremer, K. (2010) Transitioning out of sport: The psychosocial effects of collegiate athletes' career-ending injuries. *Athletic Insight*, 32(2), 1–12.

Taylor, J. and Taylor, S. (1997) *Psychological Approaches to Sports Injury Rehabilitation.* Gaithersburg, MD: Aspen.

Walsh, A. E. (2011) The relaxation response: A strategy to address stress. *International Journal of Athletic Therapy & Training*, 16(2), 20–3.

Washington-Lofren, L., Westerman, B. J., Sullivan, P. A. and Nashman, H. W. (2004) The role of the athletic trainer in the post-injury psychological recovery of collegiate athletes. *International Sports Journal*, 8, 94–104.

Weinberg, R. S. and Gould, D. (2007) *Foundations of Sport and Exercise Psychology*, 4th edn. Champaign, IL: Human Kinetics.

Wiese–Bjornstal, D. M., Smith, A. M., Shaffer, S. M. and Morrey, M. A. (1998) An integrated model of response to sport injury: Psychological and sociological dynamics. *Journal of Applied Sport Psychology*, 10, 46–69.

Williams, J. M. and Andersen, M. B. (2007) Psychosocial antecedents of sport injury and interventions for risk reduction. In G. Tenenbaum and R. Eklund (eds), *Handbook of Sport Psychology*, 3rd edn. Hoboken, NJ: Wiley, pp. 379–403.

Williams, J. M. and Scherzer, C. B. (2010) Injury risk and rehabilitation: Psychological considerations. In J. M. Williams (ed.), *Applied Sport Psychology: Personal growth to peak performance*. New York: McGraw Hill, pp. 512–41.

Yang, J. Z., Peek-Asa, C., Lowe, J., Heiden, E. and Foster, D. (2010) Social support patterns of collegiate athletes before and after injury. *Journal of Athletic Training*, 45, 372–80.

11

SPORT MEDICINE TEAM INFLUENCES IN PSYCHOLOGICAL REHABILITATION

A multidisciplinary approach

Damien Clement and Monna Arvinen-Barrow

Introduction

Injured athletes often enter the sport injury rehabilitation process with the hopes of returning to pre-injury level of fitness and performance as rapidly and safely as possible. However, research has highlighted the need to also address the psychological consequences that injured athletes often experience, to ensure their full holistic recovery (Booher and Thibodeau, 2000). Research findings to date have suggested that injured athletes' cognitive appraisal, emotional and behavioural responses to injury can have an impact on the physical and psychological recovery outcomes (for more details, see Chapter 3). In addition, the use of psychological interventions (such as goal setting, imagery, relaxation techniques, self-talk and social support) during rehabilitation can help injured athletes in dealing with a range of psychological issues that occur as a consequence of their injuries (Beneka *et al.*, 2007; Flint, 1998; Ievleva and Orlick, 1991; for more details on how to integrate psychological interventions during rehabilitation, see Chapters 5–10).

Given the importance of addressing both physical and psychological aspects of injuries during rehabilitation, there is a need to provide well-rounded and holistic care to athletes when they are injured. The process of rehabilitation, at its best, will involve a number of people working closely together for the benefit of the athlete, with the aim of ensuring a full and safe return to pre-injury (or higher) level of health, wellbeing and performance. The care provided should entail the involvement of relevant sport medicine professionals, as well as the use of sport psychologists or those equipped to provide psychological support (Green, 1992). According to Wiese-Bjornstal and Smith (1999), having a multidisciplinary team working with injured athletes is often common practice in professional sports. However, such is thought to be rarely the case amongst athletes involved in lower levels of participation. Recognising the importance of adopting a multidisciplinary approach to rehabilitation at all levels, this chapter discusses the concept of a multi-disciplinary approach to rehabilitation and demonstrates the ways in which it could be applied to various sport injury rehabilitation situations. More specifically, the chapter: (a) introduces the multidisciplinary approach to rehabilitation through primary and secondary teams, (b) details the interactions between members of the multidisciplinary team, (c) describes the process of setting up a multidisciplinary team; (d) explains the benefits of adopting a multidisciplinary approach; (e) describes the role of sport medicine professionals within this approach; (f) presents potential problems with a multidisciplinary approach; and (g) makes recommendations about the utility of a multidisciplinary approach.

The multidisciplinary approach to rehabilitation

Given the varied nature in which athletes train and compete, it is not surprising that, when injured, the rehabilitation environment and those involved in the rehabilitation process may also vary greatly. According to the psychology of injury literature, the sport medicine professionals on whom injured athletes rely during the course of their rehabilitation continue to evolve beyond the traditional physiotherapist, athletic trainer and physician (Kolt, 2000; Wiese-Bjornstal and Smith, 1999). Kolt (2000) further stated that it is not uncommon for a variety of sport medicine professionals (sport psychologists, clinical psychologists, sport therapists, massage therapists, strength and conditioning coaches and nutritionists, to name a few) to also work with injured athletes in this context, thus providing the injured athletes with access to a wide range of services to enhance, and possibly accelerate, their sport injury rehabilitation. While the notion of including sport medicine and allied health professionals within injured athletes' rehabilitation has been documented by Wiese-Bjornstal and Smith (1999), this section will introduce a development of the multidisciplinary approach to injury rehabilitation. More specifically, the notion of multidisciplinary team approach to rehabilitation will be considered through the concept of primary and secondary rehabilitation teams.

Primary and secondary rehabilitation teams

When considering rehabilitation teams, the primary rehabilitation team often consists of those sport medicine professionals who will work closely with the injured athlete from injury occurrence through the entire rehabilitation process until their successful return to the field of play. Typically, these would be the primary treatment providers (the physiotherapist/athletic trainer and the physician/orthopaedic surgeon). A number of researchers (Gordon, Potter and Ford, 1998; Gordon, Potter and Hamer, 2001; Pearson and Jones, 1992; Wiese and Weiss, 1987; Wiese, Weiss and Yukelson, 1991) are in support of the above, as they have suggested that medical professionals in regular contact with the athlete during treatment are in an ideal position to inform, educate and assist with both the psychological and physical process of injury. Indeed, it appears that members of the sport medicine team are the first to attend to injured athletes' needs (Wiese-Bjornstal and Smith, 1993) and are often available immediately after the injury occurrence. Moreover, these professionals interact with injured athletes regularly and almost exclusively during the initial stages of injury (Tunick, Clement and Etzel, 2009), at the time when the levels of pain and confusion experienced as a result of the injury by the athlete are at their worst.

In addition to the above, during rehabilitation, often those outside of primary rehabilitation team can also play a significant role in assisting the injured athletes towards successful recovery. The secondary rehabilitation team should ideally consist of a range of sport medicine and allied health professionals, as well as related others with whom injured athletes will have varying degrees of interaction throughout the course of their injury rehabilitation (Figure 11.1). It must be noted that, although the individuals who are deemed members of this team may not be directly involved in the physical treatment of the injured athlete they often

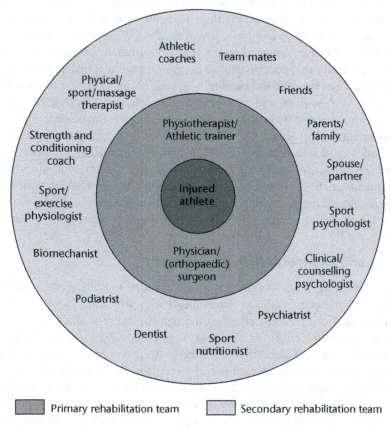

FIGURE 11.1 Structure of multidisciplinary team to rehabilitation: primary and secondary teams

contribute to the injured athlete's rehabilitation experience in myriad different ways. The individuals that should make up this team include, but are not limited to: sport nutritionist; podiatrist; dentist; sport psychologist; clinical/counselling psychologist; psychiatrist; sport/exercise physiologist; biomechanist; strength and conditioning coach; physical/sport/massage therapist; athletic coaches; parents/family; friends; spouse/partner; and team mates. Evidence exists in support of the inclusion of some of the above-mentioned professionals and significant others in facilitating sport injury rehabilitation process. For example, the role of sport psychologists in injury rehabilitation has been highlighted as important but very seldom is such used to its full capacity (see, for example, Arvinen-Barrow, Hemmings, Weigand, Becker and Booth, 2007; Arvinen-Barrow, Penny, Hemmings and Corr, 2010; Brewer, 1998; Clement, Granquist and Arvinen-Barrow, 2013; Heaney, Green, Rostron and Walker, 2012; Larson, Starkey and Zaichkowsky, 1996). The role of coaches has also received some attention in the literature. However, the usefulness of research findings is equivocal. It appears that coaches may serve multiple roles (teachers, parental figures, disciplinarians) and therefore may have both direct and indirect influences over the injury rehabilitation and subsequent playing status once returning back to sport (Tunick *et al.*, 2009; Yang, Peek-Asa, Lowe, Heiden and Foster, 2010). The importance of parents/family, friends, spouses and partners has also been recognised in the literature, as a number of studies have found them to be a significant source of different forms of social support during injury rehabilitation (for example, Johnston and Carroll, 1998; Yang *et al.*, 2010; for more details see Chapter 9). In a similar manner, support from team mates or other athletes who have since recovered from similar injuries or the use of performance-enhancement groups consisting of injured athletes has also been found to be beneficial (Clement, Shannon and Connole, 2011; Yang *et al.*, 2010).

> Medical professionals in regular contact with the athlete (that is, the primary team) during treatment are in an ideal position to inform, educate and assist with both the psychological and physical process of injury. Whilst members of the secondary team may not be directly involved in the physical treatment of the injured athlete they often contribute to the injured athlete's rehabilitation experience in numerous ways.

Interactions within and between the different members of the rehabilitation teams

Despite the obvious distinction between the two rehabilitation teams, the roles of the various members of each team may interact and intertwine in a number of ways. Some of the roles may be direct (that is, the ways in which family members and spouse/partner can facilitate recovery), whereas others may be more indirect (that is, the podiatrist may influence the rehabilitation process through the

physiotherapist/athletic trainer). Moreover, the strength and nature of these relationships may change across the rehabilitation stages, depending on the injured
athlete's needs and the athlete's personal and situational factors. For example, the
type of injury (a personal factor) can impact the extent of tangible support an
athlete may need from those close to them. In a similar manner, an athlete with
recurrent injuries may need direct or indirect involvement from various members
of the sport medicine team (a situational factor). For instance, an athlete with
recurrent problems with shin splints and the physiotherapist/athletic trainer with
whom they are working may need to consult a podiatrist and/or a biomechanist
to ensure the underlying cause for the shin splints will be treated appropriately. In
a similar manner, an athlete may require regular consultations with a sport psychologist to deal with self-confidence issues that may have amplified as a result of the
injury. Moreover, access (or lack of) to appropriate support from sport medicine
and allied health professionals may also change the roles and relationships of those
involved with the injured athlete on a day to day basis.

One of the ways in which these relationships could be examined is through the
use of sociograms. A sociogram is a tool to measure social cohesion by disclosing
affiliations and attractions within a group (Weinberg and Gould, 2011) but it could
also be modified to sport injury rehabilitation settings with the aim of establishing
and gaining clarity of the roles, relationships and interactions between the different
members involved in the rehabilitation process (Figure 11.2). It is also believed that
a sociogram could be used to highlight the impact (direct/indirect) that different
members of the multidisciplinary team may have on injured athletes. It is hoped
that this increased awareness could help facilitate improved communication and
consequently build trust and rapport among all those involved in the process.

Setting up a multidisciplinary team: the process

In most cases, injured athletes, depending on their sporting level, would have a
primary rehabilitation team in place. This assumption is based on the fact that it is
common knowledge that physiotherapists/athletic trainers and physicians are all
intricately involved in the care and ultimate rehabilitation of the injured athlete
(Wiese-Bjornstal and Smith, 1993). The members of the secondary team, on the
other hand, are often sport medicine and allied health professionals and relevant
(significant) others who have been used on occasions but have not been traditionally considered part of the rehabilitation team.

However, in the hope of establishing a secondary rehabilitation team, the phys-
iotherapist/athletic trainer who will serve as the point person for the injured
athlete's rehabilitation programme will first determine who needs to be involved
from the sport medicine and allied health professionals and significant others previously mentioned. This decision should be made in consultation with the physician
and possibly the injured athlete. Once a potential list has been generated and the
merits for the involvement of each of these individuals have been thoroughly given
consideration, the physiotherapist/athletic trainer will need to contact each

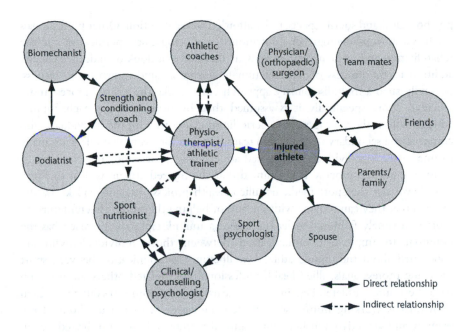

FIGURE 11.2 An example of a sociogram in injury rehabilitation setting

individual to determine their level of interest in being involved as a member of a secondary rehabilitation team for a specific athlete. Assuming that each potential member agrees to participate, their roles and responsibilities within the secondary rehabilitation team should be thoroughly explained. Following this, it is advised that a meeting should be organised to formalise and identify (and introduce in person, if possible) all members of both the primary and secondary rehabilitation teams. This meeting will serve three purposes: (1) to introduce members to each other; (2) to educate each member about the possible resources at the injured athlete's disposal; and (3) enable all members to establish and come to an agreement on a referral protocol for the involved injured athlete. Finally, it would seem imperative that the injured athlete be introduced to all members of the secondary rehabilitation team.

Benefits of multidisciplinary approach to rehabilitation

Adopting the multidisciplinary approach to injury rehabilitation has the potential to offer a number of benefits to injured athletes. Firstly, this approach allows injured athletes to be exposed to a holistic approach to injury rehabilitation. Using this approach could potentially enable injured athletes to be exposed to a rehabilitation protocol that no longer focuses solely on the physical aspect of injury rehabilitation but instead offers opportunities for once neglected areas, such as the psychological and social aspects, to be afforded some attention. Other professionals (such as a sport psychologist or a nutritionist) can bring a new perspective into the rehabilitation and, as such, offer athletes an alternative outlook or, indeed, a needed addition to the process of rehabilitation to ensure a rapid return to full fitness. Secondly, such a multidisciplinary approach could make the referral process more efficient. More specifically, it is assumed that, by using this approach, injured athletes will, at the very least, have periodic interactions with the individuals who comprise the secondary rehabilitation team. Thus, in the event that referral is made to one of these individuals, the injured athlete may be less resistant to or apprehensive about the process. It is assumed that the injured athlete will, at the very least, have met the sport medicine/allied health professional and will know the services that they can provide with the aim of helping them (the athlete) return to sport in a timely fashion. Finally, the use of a multidisciplinary approach has the potential to improve communication between those individuals who are concerned about the injured athlete's wellbeing. Communication between sport medicine professionals, allied health professionals and related others, all of whom have the injured athlete's best interest at heart, can sometimes be difficult if each individual is working from a solitary view. However, with the use both of the primary and secondary rehabilitation teams all members should, it is hoped, be 'on the same page' with regard to the injured athlete. It is anticipated that increased interaction between both teams will not only promote the aforementioned holistic approach but will open, and ultimately improve, lines of communication. For example, coaches (members of the secondary rehabilitation team) could be consulted by the physiotherapist/athletic trainer (members of the primary rehabilitation team) about sport-specific drills and exercises which could be incorporated into an athlete's rehabilitation programme as he/she readies themselves for return to play. By doing this, the coach would be kept abreast of the athlete's progress and the physiotherapist/athletic trainer would be able to incorporate appropriate sport specific exercises to prepare the athlete for his/her return to the field of play.

A multidisciplinary approach in action

When I was injured for the second time during the season, I must admit I was a bit blasé about the whole thing. I didn't really follow the physio's instructions, and I know I was a pain to live with. I was lucky my girlfriend did not leave me because of how I was back then. But then one day I got dragged into a team meeting, and got a big telling off, and the coaches were like, what are you doing, and I thought oh no, and then from then on end I was sort of a bit more . . . engaged . . . I mean I wanted to know what was going on, and the team physio, coach and the psych people all helped me to understand the full picture . . . So I snapped back into reality from there on really.

(Professional rugby union player, cited in Arvinen-Barrow, 2009)

Role of sport medicine professionals

As highlighted in previous chapters of this book, research findings to date have provided support for the use of goal setting, imagery, relaxation, self-talk and social support as a means of assisting injured athletes with the range of injury-related emotional issues they may experience. Thus, given the increased importance of addressing both the physical and psychological aspects of injury rehabilitation, members of the primary rehabilitation team should take a leading role in the incorporation of a psychological component within injury rehabilitation, since a trained and qualified sport psychologist may not always be available to injured athletes.

It has been suggested that sport medicine professionals who deal with athletes on a day-to-day basis play an integral part of the sport injury rehabilitation process and that they are best suited to inform, educate and assist injured athletes with the psychological and physical processes of injury (Pearson and Jones, 1992; Wiese and Weiss, 1987; Wiese et al., 1991). As the sport medicine professional's job often involves working with injured athletes on a one-to-one basis, the likelihood of effective communication, building trust and rapport with the athletes will be increased, subsequently having the potential to facilitate greater levels of rehabilitation adherence and treatment compliance, to increase motivation and ultimately having a positive impact on the overall recovery process (see, for example, Arvinen-Barrow, 2009).

Kolt (2003) supported this assertion by stating that sport medicine professionals are best suited to provide psychological assistance for injured athletes for three main reasons:

1. Psychological issues which often present themselves as a result of injury are often discussed in conjunction with physical aspects of rehabilitation (Kolt, 2003);
2. The treatment and rehabilitation of injured athletes typically involves touch, which can often facilitate athletes opening up to their sport medicine professional about psychological issues in their recovery (Nathan, 1999);
3. Existing studies suggest that athletes themselves feel that sport medicine professionals are in an ideal situation to address the psychological aspects of injury (Larson et al., 1996; Wiese and Weiss, 1987; Wiese et al., 1991).

Based on the aforementioned, it appears that sport medicine professionals are well suited to provide psychological support to injured athletes, owing to their adjacent position with the athlete during the recovery process. Moreover, sport medicine professionals also have a substantial role in providing both direct and indirect psychological support to injured athletes, to ensure full recovery.

Recommendations for promoting and using a multidisciplinary approach

It is suggested that, in the absence of an access to a sport psychologist, sport medicine professionals are not only in an ideal position to address psychological aspects of sport injuries but are also best positioned to facilitate a multidisciplinary approach to sport injury rehabilitation. This section includes a number of recommendations on how sport medicine professionals can not only incorporate a multidisciplinary approach to rehabilitation but also address the psychological component in their work with injured athletes. As such sport medicine professionals should:

- know their role in cultivating a multidisciplinary approach to rehabilitation;
- recognise the importance of significant others (such as team mates, friends, family/parents, spouse) in ensuring a holistic approach to recovery;
- demonstrate increased awareness of psychological issues which athletes may experience as a result of athletic injuries;
- think about ways in which psychology could be integrated into rehabilitation as part of the process rather than an addition to it;
- continue to seek out additional training in the area of psychological rehabilitation;
- know professional boundaries and competencies;
- know when and to whom to refer athletes;
- have access to a network of other sport medicine and allied health professionals and related others.

Know their role in cultivating a multidisciplinary approach to rehabilitation

As the individuals who play a leading role in the treatment and rehabilitation of injured athletes, sport medicine professionals should understand that they alone cannot provide all the services these individuals may require. Part of ensuring full recovery, both psychologically and physically, is to ensure that all areas affecting the injury recovery (nutritional, biomechanical and social) are addressed appropriately by relevant professionals. Thus, the onus should be on the primary treatment providers to attempt to involve as many other sport medicine and allied health professionals and related others as needed in athletes' treatment and rehabilitation.

Recognise the importance of significant others in ensuring a holistic approach to recovery

As the above-mentioned significant others typically spend a considerable amount of time with the injured athlete, they are in a position to impact athletes' thinking, emotions and behaviour. As such, it is imperative for the members of the primary rehabilitation team to have an awareness of those individuals and to have the ability to educate them about the importance of their role in the athlete's recovery.

Demonstrate increased awareness of psychological issues which athletes may experience as a result of athletic injuries

Sport medicine professionals, by virtue of their interactions with injured athletes, should be acutely aware that the ramifications of athletic injuries go beyond the physical domain. Furthermore, injured athletes, depending on the severity of their injuries, often experience a range of thoughts, feelings, emotions and behaviours, some of which can have a negative effect on injury recovery (see, for example, Fisher and Wrisberg, 2006). By demonstrating increased awareness of the potential psychological issues that athletes may experience, sport medicine professionals could possibly help facilitate the incorporation of a psychological component within rehabilitation programmes.

Think about ways in which psychology could be integrated into rehabilitation as part of the process rather than an addition to it

While it is acknowledged and appreciated that sport medicine professionals are not traditionally trained to integrate psychology into rehabilitation, they should be encouraged to start thinking of ways of promoting a more holistic approach to rehabilitation. Sport medicine professionals may want to consider asking questions related to injured athletes' thoughts, feelings, emotions and behaviours as a result of injury. In addition, they should seek to gain an understanding of injured athlete's expectations of the rehabilitation process, as these should be in line with those of the sport medicine professionals (Clement *et al.*, 2012). By asking these questions, sport medicine professionals would be taking a step in the right direction with regards to integrating a psychological component appropriately within injury reha-bilitation. More importantly, asking these questions could also help to build trust and rapport between the athlete and the sport medicine professional, as well as rais-ing the injured athlete's awareness of the importance of the psychological aspect of sport injury.

Continue to seek out additional training in the area of psychological rehabilitation

As mentioned above, sport medicine professionals are not trained in psychological aspects of sport injuries and how to use psychological skills and techniques in their work. However, as they are often required to address psychological issues in their work, they should seek out avenues, such as continuing education courses, confer-ences, lectures or training modules, that could help increase their knowledge in this area (Arvinen-Barrow, Hemmings, Becker and Booth, 2008).

Know professional boundaries and competencies

Although sport medicine professionals should be encouraged to demonstrate increased awareness with regard to psychological issues, it must be reiterated that they should strive to continue to provide services that are consistent with their training and level of competence.

Know when and to whom to refer athletes

Sport medicine professionals, at the very least, should be able to recognise the signs and symptoms of psychological issues that should be referred to trained professionals (Arvinen-Barrow *et al.*, 2010). Of greater importance, sport medicine professionals should possess the ability to acutely communicate the need for a referral to the injured athlete and the appropriate sport medicine professionals and allied health professionals required and to be able to facilitate the referral process in a timely fashion.

Have access to a network of other sport medicine and allied health professionals and related others

Sport medicine professionals should also develop a network of trusted referrals that they can utilise in times of need. Developing these professional relationships will increase the ease at which these individuals can become involved in a multidisciplinary team.

When dealing with psychological issues sport medicine professionals should:

- know their role in cultivating a multidisciplinary approach to rehabilitation;
- be able to recognise the importance of significant others;
- be able to demonstrate increased awareness of psychological issues with which athletes may present;
- think about ways in which psychology could be integrated into physical rehabilitation;
- continue to seek out additional training in the area;
- engage in networks with other relevant professionals and related others;
- know their professional boundaries and competencies;
- know when and to whom to refer athletes when deemed necessary.

Possible problems in multidisciplinary approach to rehabilitation

Despite the previously mentioned benefits which could be derived from a multidisciplinary approach to injury rehabilitation, some concerns with regard to sport medicine professionals' ability to effectively facilitate this process must be taken into consideration. These problems may include: (a) a lack of awareness of the sport medicine professional's prominent role in the multidisciplinary approach to rehabilitation; (b) the sport medicine professional's lack of confidence and ability to take the lead in a multidisciplinary approach to rehabilitation (for example, Hamson-Utley, Martin and Walters, 2008; Kamphoff *et al.*, 2010); (c) the sport medicine professional's lack of appropriate training and understanding of the importance of the psychological aspects of sport injury rehabilitation (Arvinen-Barrow *et al.*, 2010; Heaney *et al.*, 2012); (d) the sport medicine professional's lack of appropriate referral procedures and skills in making referrals (Larson *et al.*, 1996); and (e) the sport medicine professional's lack of access to other relevant allied health professionals (Arvinen-Barrow *et al.*, 2007; Clement *et al.*, 2013).

Conclusion

Despite the various innovations made to training philosophies and equipment, athletes at various levels of competition continue to sustain injuries which can limit, and in some cases prevent, their subsequent athletic participation temporarily or for a prolonged period of time. While the treatment of the physical aspects of these injuries have typically been the main focus of traditional rehabilitation programmes, sport medicine professionals are beginning to give increasing attention to the psychological consequences of injuries. Thus, the use of a holistic approach to injury rehabilitation is becoming increasingly common and should be advocated more widely across varying rehabilitation settings. Consequently, it is suggested that a multidisciplinary team composed of sport medicine professionals, allied health professionals and related others should apply. This chapter has provided details regarding the process of setting up a multidisciplinary team, the role of the sport medicine professional within such a team and the many benefits which can be derived from using this approach. Finally, possible problems were presented which could arise with a multidisciplinary approach in addition to recommendations to promote the use of such teams.

CASE STUDY

Devin is a 20-year-old African American collegiate soccer player who suffered an anterior cruciate ligament injury to his right knee 16 months ago and has since returned back to field in full fitness as scheduled. However, just over a month ago, Devin suffered his second anterior cruciate ligament injury to the same knee. Upon the diagnosis of the injury, Devin's surgery was scheduled and completed within three weeks. Since both injuries occurred at college, Devin will once again be completing his rehabilitation under the guidance of his college's team physician and athletic trainer. Despite the fact that Devin was able to rehabilitate his first injury successfully, he has admitted to his family, team mates and girlfriend that he lacks confidence in his rehabilitation programme. He reports that having sustained the same injury again has created major doubts in his mind with regards to the skills and competence level of his athletic trainer.

Devin also reports anxiety-related symptoms, which he feels are linked to his impending rehabilitation. Devin has also admitted that, on a number of occasions, he has been using alcohol to help him deal with the pain and potential lost season. 'I mean I am just so frustrated about the thought of not playing this season … this could really end my career as a professional before it has even started … and getting drunk just helps me forget for a while.' He further admits that his eating habits have become very inconsistent, owing to his lack of mobility. Devin has also been interacting with his team mates a lot less than usual and is choosing to be by himself. He has even mentioned that the fact that he is an African American at a predominately white college is beginning to bother him. In fact, he is the only ethnic minority player on his team and he now feels like an 'outsider' within the team and in university life as a whole.

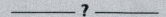

1. What multidisciplinary team members would the athletic trainer/physiotherapist want to incorporate into this athlete's rehabilitation programme?
2. What are some of the psychological issues the athlete is presenting with that may go beyond the athletic trainer/physiotherapist's competence level?
3. As an athletic trainer/physiotherapist, please explain how you would proceed in dealing with this athlete?

References

Arvinen-Barrow, M. (2009) *Psychological rehabilitation from sport injury: Issues in the training and development of chartered physiotherapists.* (Doctoral dissertation). University of Northampton. Retrieved from http://nectar.northampton.ac.uk/2456/

Arvinen-Barrow, M., Hemmings, B., Becker, C. A. and Booth, L. (2008) Sport psychology education: A preliminary survey into chartered physiotherapists' preferred methods of training delivery. *Journal of Sport Rehabilitation,* 17(4), 399–412.

Arvinen-Barrow, M., Hemmings, B., Weigand, D. A., Becker, C. A. and Booth, L. (2007) Views of chartered physiotherapists on the psychological content of their practice: A national follow-up survey in the United Kingdom. *Journal of Sport Rehabilitation,* 16, 111–21.

Arvinen-Barrow, M., Penny, G., Hemmings, B. and Corr, S. (2010) UK chartered physiotherapists' personal experiences in using psychological interventions with injured athletes: an interpretative phenomenological analysis. *Psychology of Sport and Exercise,* 11(1), 58–66.

Beneka, A., Malliou, P., Bebetsos, E., Gioftsidou, A., Pafis, G. and Godolias, G. (2007) Appropriate counselling techniques for specific components of the rehabilitation plan: A review of the literature. *Physical Training.* Retrieved from http://ejmas.com/pt/2007pt/ptart_beneka_0707.html

Booher, J. M. and Thibodeau, G. A. (2000) *Athletic Injury Assessment*. Boston, MA: McGraw Hill.

Brewer, B. W. (1998) Psychological applications in clinical sports medicine: current status and future directions. *Journal of Clinical Psychology in Medical Settings*, 5(1), 93–102.

Clement, D., Granquist, M. and Arvinen-Barrow, M. (2013) Psychosocial aspects of athletic injuries as perceived by athletic trainers. *Journal of Athletic Training*.

Clement, D., Hamson-Utley, J. J., Arvinen-Barrow, M., Kamphoff, C., Zakrajsek, R. A. and Martin, S. B. (2012) College athletes' expectations about injury rehabilitation with an athletic trainer. *International Journal of Athletic Therapy & Training*, 17(4), 18–27.

Clement, D., Shannon, V. R. and Connole, I. J. (2011) Performance enhancement groups for injured athletes. *International Journal of Athletic Therapy & Training*, 16(3), 34–6.

Fisher, L. A. and Wrisberg, C. A. (2006) What athletic training students want to know about sport psychology. *Athletic Therapy Today*, 11(3), 32–3.

Flint, F. A. (1998) Specialized psychological interventions In F. A. Flint (ed.), *Psychology of Sport Injury*. Leeds: Human Kinetics, pp. 29–50.

Gordon, S., Potter, M. and Ford, I. W. (1998) Toward a psychoeducational curriculum for training sport-injury rehabilitation personnel. *Journal of Applied Sport Psychology*, 10, 140–56.

Gordon, S., Potter, M. and Hamer, P. (2001) The role of the physiotherapist and sport therapist. In J. Crossman (ed.), *Coping with Sport Injuries: Psychological strategies for rehabilitation*. New York: Oxford University Press, pp. 62–82.

Green, L. B. (1992) The use of imagery in the rehabilitation of injured athletes. *The Sport Psychologist*, 6, 416–28.

Hamson-Utley, J. J., Martin, S. and Walters, J. (2008) Athletic trainers' and physical therapists' perceptions of the effectiveness of psychological skills within sport injury rehabilitation programs. *Journal of Athletic Training*, 43(3), 258–64.

Heaney, C., Green, A. J. K., Rostron, C. L. and Walker, N. (2012) A Qualitative and Quantitative Investigation of the Psychology Content of UK Physiotherapy Education Programs. *Journal of Physical Therapy Education*, 26(3), 48–56.

Ievleva, L. and Orlick, T. (1991) Mental links to enhanced healing: An exploratory study. *The Sport Psychologist*, 5, 25–40.

Johnston, L. H. and Carroll, D. (1998) The context of emotional responses to athletic injury: A qualitative analysis. *Journal of Sport Rehabilitation*, 7, 206–20.

Kamphoff, C., Hamson-Utley, J. J., Antoine, B., Knutson, B., Thomae, J. and Hoenig, C. (2010) Athletic training students' perceptions of the importance and effectiveness of psychological skills within sport injury rehabilitation. *Athletic Training Education Journal*, 5(3), 109–16.

Kolt, G. S. (2000) Doing sport psychology with injured athletes. In M. B. Andersen (ed.), *Doing Sport Psychology*. Champaign, IL: Human Kinetics, pp. 223–36.

Kolt, G. S. (2003) Psychology of injury and rehabilitation. In G. S. Kolt and L. Snyder-Mackler (eds), *Physical Therapies in Sport and Exercise*. London: Churchill Livingstone, pp. 165–83.

Larson, G. A., Starkey, C. and Zaichkowsky, L. D. (1996) Psychological aspects of athletic injuries as perceived by athletic trainers. *The Sport Psychologist*, 10, 37–47.

Nathan, B. (1999) *Touch and Emotion in Manual Therapy*. London: Churchill Livingstone.

Pearson, L. and Jones, G. (1992) Emotional effects of sports injuries: Implications for physiotherapists. *Physiotherapy*, 78(10), 762–70.

Tunick, R., Clement, D. and Etzel, E. F. (2009) Counseling injured and disabled student-athletes: a guide for understanding and intervention. In E. F. Etzel (ed.), *Counseling and Psychological Services for College Student-athletes*. Morgantown, WV: Fitness Information Technology.

Weinberg, R. S. and Gould, D. (2011) *Foundations of Sport and Exercise Psychology*. Champaign, IL: Human Kinetics.

Wiese, D. M. and Weiss, M. R. (1987) Psychological rehabilitation and physical injury: Implications for the sportsmedicine team. *The Sport Psychologist*, 1, 318–30.

Wiese, D. M., Weiss, M. R. and Yukelson, D. P. (1991) Sport psychology in the training room: A survey of athletic trainers. *The Sport Psychologist*, 5, 15–24.

Wiese-Bjornstal, D. M. and Smith, A. M. (1993) Counseling strategies for enhanced recovery of injured athletes within a team approach. In D. Pargman (ed.), *Psychological Bases of Sport Injuries*. Morgantown, WV: Fitness Information Technology, pp. 149–82.

Wiese-Bjornstal, D. M. and Smith, A. M. (1999) Counseling strategies for enhanced recovery of injured athletes within team approach. In D. Pargman (ed.), *Psychological Bases of Sport Injuries*, 2nd edn. Morgantown, WV: Fitness Information Technology, pp. 125–55.

Yang, J. Z., Peek-Asa, C., Lowe, J., Heiden, E. and Foster, D. (2010) Social support patterns of collegiate athletes before and after injury. *Journal of Athletic Training*, 45, 372–80.

12

USING A PSYCHOLOGICAL MODEL AND COUNSELLING SKILLS IN SPORT INJURY REHABILITATION

Julie A. Waumsley and Jonathan Katz

Introduction

> Harry is a 27-year-old male basketball player. His coach suggested he see a sport psychologist because he has recently recovered from an elbow injury but can't seem to get back into training properly. He's worked with a sports psychologist on motivation issues and has used goal setting, self-talk and imagery but is still having problems. He keeps avoiding the hard training sessions and wants to be on his own more than he used to be. He has said more often of late that none of the psychological work he's doing is making any difference.

Harry's quote highlights several issues that present for consideration over and above the obvious. First, there is persistence avoidance to training following injury recovery indicating the need for further in-depth work. Second, the athlete acknowledges that he is experiencing social withdrawal. Thirdly, there is a sense of persistent low mood accompanying the negative language in this athlete's presentation.

Working with the unsaid, implied issues that lie between the athlete and what he/she is presenting requires an ability to recognise and work within the process. Further, a willingness to gain a depth of understanding of issues such as personality characteristics, emotional reactions, coping mechanisms, past behaviours impacting current ones and thinking patterns is helpful. Moreover, recognising clinical features within an athlete presentation, such as anxiety, depression, and post-traumatic stress disorder, and the ways in which these might manifest in an athlete following injury will require the professional knowledge that underpins a process of working within a trustworthy working alliance. This therapeutic '-

difference' from sport psychology echoes a way of working that various models of counselling and therapy underpin and define in contrasting ways, which makes it difficult to offer just one definition.

McLeod (2011) offers that counselling is 'an activity that takes place when someone who is troubled *invites* and allows another person to enter into a particular kind of relationship with them' (p.12). Given that injured athletes are often 'troubled' by the changes their injury imposes on them, the philosophy and underpinning of the approach of the professional applied work offered may be broader or different from that of a cognitive behavioural approach to mental skill straining, which is often the adopted approach by sport psychologists (Katz and Hemmings, 2009). Within counselling, the psychodynamic, cognitive behavioural and humanistic approaches are generally recognised as the three primary models. A counsellor's applied work will often be underpinned by one such approach, although it is true to say that the integrative approach, where several models integrate to form one theory (Katz and Hemmings, 2009) has been adopted by many practitioners.

This chapter offers an account of the process of working within an injury-and-rehabilitation environment. More specifically, the chapter demonstrates the usefulness of using a psychological model and counselling skills in sport injury rehabilitation context. The chapter: (a) offers a summary of the key theoretical and applied models that underpin a counselling approach; (b) introduces the key counselling skills deemed as useful in sport injury rehabilitation context, c) offers an account of the process of working within an injury and rehabilitation environment, and (d) discusses some of the key issues to consider when using counselling skills with injured athletes.

For the purposes of clarity within this chapter, the term 'practitioner' is generically used in places to avoid confusion between the terms 'sports psychologist', 'counsellor', or 'therapist'. In addition, the term 'athlete' will be used to avoid confusion between 'patient' or 'client'. The concept of 'relationship' in this context refers to the therapeutic element of the work where there is an unconditional, non-judgemental and congruently empathic respect for the athlete and the 'process' that occurs in the space in between the content of what is being verbally articulated and what is being experienced by the athlete internally.

It's great to work with a counsellor and to also know that she's working with the psychologist. I really feel that she 'gets' me. I can't really talk about this stuff to anyone else for all sorts of reasons. People will think I'm a freak or disgusting, or both. I'm scared that sports people will think I'm not worth investing in any more. My counsellor just accepts me and it's funny, but we don't talk much about food; we talk about what it all means so that makes me feel that I'm not so much a disgusting freak but more someone who is worthwhile listening to. My counsellor helps me to understand why I do what I do. She doesn't invest in my performance at all and that's refreshing. I feel much more motivated and unburdened after I have seen my counsellor.

(Jill, female 15-year-old gymnast)

Theoretical approaches

The psychoanalytical/psychodynamic approach

Psychoanalysis is defined as a theory of the mind or personality, a method of investigation of unconscious processes and a method of treatment (Freud, 1949). Much of Sigmund Freud's theorising was on the development of personality and of the consequences of what he regarded as abnormal development, with the emphasis on the unconscious. This is the notion that unconscious motivations and needs have a role in determining behaviour. Freud's theory might perhaps be divided into three main parts: a description of the mind or psyche, a description of the development of the psyche and a description of the way in which the psyche defends itself. Freud's topographic model of the psyche view the mind as having three levels of consciousness: the conscious, the pre-conscious and the unconscious. He saw the conscious as everything we are aware of. The pre-conscious is the area of the mind containing thoughts and ideas which are available to recall but are currently 'at the back of ones mind'. This is quite different from the unconscious, which Freud saw as holding all the early thoughts and feelings that might cause anxiety, conflict or pain, and which are the motivating factors, out of awareness and not generally accessible, that drive behaviour. The id functions at an unconscious level, driving primitive needs and is 'controlled' by the ego. The superego brings a moral sense to behaviour. Freud's complex view of the 'inner self' describes the ego as battling against the id and the superego; the 'three aspects of 'self' (Jacobs, 1991). Freud believed that personality develops through a stage theory of psychosexual development, as shown in Table 12.1.

TABLE 12.1 Freud's stages of psychosexual development

Psychosexual stage	Time frame (years)	Behaviour
Oral	Birth to 12–18 months	Child is focused on oral pleasures (sucking)
Anal	12–18 months to 3 years	Pleasure is on eliminating and retaining faeces, learning control and stimulation
Phallic	3–6	Pleasure zone becomes the genitals. Oedipus complex develops (boys develop unconscious desires for their mother). More recent psychoanalysis's describe the same process for girls as the Electra complex
Latency	7–12	Sexual urges remain repressed. Children interact mostly with same-sex peers
Genital	12–18	Primary focus of pleasure is genitals and sexual urges are awakened. Adolescents direct their sexual urges to opposite sex peers

In Freud's stages of psychosexual development he contends that various crises are resolved at each stage, leading to a healthy or unhealthy personality. If these crises get 'stuck' at a specific stage they will be apparent and manifest in adult behaviour. Consistent with this, the concept of anxiety is central to Freud's theory. According to Freud, the dynamics of all human behaviour were conflicts between the expression of and inhibition of desires and needs. To deal with this conflict between inhibitions and desires and needs, Freud developed a series of defence mechanisms, such as denial, repression, projection, regression, which would prevent immediate goal gratification and resolve the conflict by transferring it into a socially acceptable form. Thus, when anxiety cannot be dealt with by realistic methods that are socially acceptable, the ego calls on various defence mechanisms to release the resultant build-up of tensions. These defence mechanisms defy, alter or falsify reality, work unconsciously and are not immediately obvious to ourselves or other people.

Working with individuals in a psychoanalytical way will involve working with the unconscious drives through free association and dream work, when the analyst interprets what is being said to make sense of it to the athlete. Central to this approach are the concepts of transference and countertransference. Transference refers to the way our athletes relate to us based on experiences with those who cared for them in their formative years. Thus, they bring with them expectations and assumptions based on their experiences of life that will influence the way they perceive the practitioner (Gray, 2007). The practitioner can begin to learn about these previous experiences by listening to what the athlete is saying and by noticing the ways in which they relate to us. Countertransference can be useful in learning about how athletes relate to others but the practitioner must be sufficiently skilled and self-aware to, sometimes painfully, recognise some feelings within a therapeutic alliance do not belong to the athlete but to the practitioner's own unresolved difficulties (Gray, 2007).

The cognitive behavioural approach

Behaviour therapy evolved from the theories of human learning (Hough, 2006). However, 'pure' behaviourism left little room for any cognitive aspects associated with human behaviour. Thus, taking note of both behaviour and cognition led on to a cognitive behavioural approach. The Freudian approach was emphatic in the belief that unconscious forces and unseen impulses were at the root of most human problems. To deal with this, it was necessary to shed light on these hidden areas of personality in therapy. In contrast, the behavioural approach adopts an alternative philosophy. Within the behavioural approach, the focus is placed directly on the athlete's inappropriate behaviour and the associated contingencies reinforcing this behaviour. Thus, behavioural change is central within behavioural therapy, with an emphasis on targeting undesirable behaviour adapting the athlete to promote appropriate behavioural change.

Ivan Pavlov (1849–1936) is perhaps the most well-known behavioural psychologist. His work conditioned dogs to salivate at the sound of a bell that they had learned to associate with food, a sequence of events Pavlov called the 'conditioned response' and the concept of 'classical conditioning'. Watson (1878–1958) contended that conditioning could also be reversed through unconditioning and Thorndike (1874–1949) suggested the 'law of effect' when, if a response to a specific stimulus is followed by a reward, the bond between the stimulus and response will be strengthened; if the response is followed by a negative outcome, the bond will be weakened. According to Thorndike, therefore, behaviour is dependent upon its consequences, which may be either reward or punishment. Skinner (1904–1990) developed Thorndike's law of effect further to suggest that 'operant conditioning' reinforces reward or punishment and the principle of reinforcement is important to both behavioural change and maintenance of appropriate behaviour.

Ellis (1913–2007) and Beck (born 1921) started their careers as psychoanalysts but came to believe that cognitions (thoughts, attitudes, beliefs, and so on) played an important role in emotional and behavioural consequences or outcomes. Ellis's approach, currently known as rational emotive behaviour therapy, is operationalised using the A-B-C model, with A being the activating event, B being the belief and C being the emotional and behavioural consequence. Ellis argued that emotional difficulties are a consequence of 'distorted thinking' and problems occur when people's interpretation of situations and events around them is excessively biased from the 'reality' of those situations or events. More rational (realistic) belief statements allow a person to cope with relationship difficulties in a more constructive and balanced fashion with their interpretation being consistent with 'the facts'.

Beck suggests some commonalities between cognitive and behavioural approaches: 'both employ a structured, problem solving or symptom reduction approach with a highly active therapy style and both stress the "here-and-now" rather than making speculative reconstruction of the patient's childhood relationships and early family relationships' (Beck, 1976: 321). The cognitive behavioural approach concentrates on the stimulus, the cognitions and emotions and the behavioural outcome. Three key features of this approach are its problem-solving delivery style, with change in focus from interpretative in the psychoanalytic model to working collaboratively with clients, a respect for scientific values and a close attention to the cognitive processes through which people monitor, control and mediate their behaviour.

Kelly (1905–1967) has also been categorised as a cognitive theorist. Kelly sought to investigate the world as constructed by the individual. Personal construct psychology is concerned with the ways in which clients represent or view their own experiences rather than seeing them as victims of impulses and defences. Kelly's therapeutic process is concerned with helping the client to find appropriate or useful constructs rather than to be concerned with diagnosis and categorisation. This approach aims to help clients to expand and articulate meanings by which they construct a sense of self. Becoming aware of their personal constructs and thereby of their ways of thinking and feeling, leads to modifying behaviour in a similar way to the aims of cognitive behavioural therapy (CBT).

Working with athletes using a cognitive behavioural therapeutic approach will often involve establishing a rapport and building the therapeutic alliance, explaining rationale for treatment, assessing the problem, setting goals and targets primarily for cognitive and behavioural change and monitoring progress. Some ways of executing this might be through challenging irrational beliefs, reframing issues using cognitive restructuring techniques, scaling feelings, *in vivo* exposure and homework assignments (for more details on how CBT has been applied in the sport injury context, see the description of Wiese-Bjornstal, Smith, Shaffer and Morrey's (1998) integrated model of response to athletic injury and rehabilitation process presented in Chapter 3 and Chapters 5–8 on different psychological interventions).

The humanistic approach

Perhaps the most well-known humanist or phenomenological theorist is Carl Rogers (1902–1987). In Roger's view, behaviour is typically an attempt by human beings to meet their own needs as they perceive them (Rogers, 1980). The emphasis of this approach to counselling is on the athlete's perceptions as determinants of their actions. Rogers abandoned specific motivational constructs and viewed individuals as functioning as an organised whole. He suggested, 'there is one central force of energy in the human organism; that is a function of the whole organism rather than some portion of it; and that is perhaps best conceptualised as a tendency toward fulfilment, toward actualisation, toward the maintenance and enhancement of the organism, (Rogers, 1963: 6). According to Rogers, people who are self-actualising are fully functioning individuals who are open to new experiences and trust their feelings rather than being threatened by them. Within this approach, self-actualisation is seen as the fundamental motivation and underpins the notion that athletes have the necessary resources for dealing with their own problems effectively. Thus, athletes are encouraged, in a non-directive way, to explore their own solutions to their issues or problems.

Working with athletes using this approach will be underpinned by what Rogers called the 'core conditions' of empathy, unconditional positive regard and congruence, without which self-actualisation will not be achieved. The core conditions allow a therapeutic relationship of trust and non-judgement to develop, within which the process of work between athlete and practitioner allows the space for self-actualisation to be realised. The development of this therapeutic relationship requires the use of various counselling skills, which are highlighted in the next section of this chapter.

The integrative approach

There are many integrative approaches that underpin athlete work in different ways (see, for example Clarkson, 2007; Lapworth, Sills and Fish, 2007; Moursund and Erskine, 2004). However, integrating the three primary models is suggested as one way of working and it is attractive because this allows not only to work with presenting issues but to better understand why past experiences impact on current mechanisms of coping and behaviour, and to do so within a relationship or 'working alliance' that is conducive to positive change. To illustrate this, a model is suggested in Figure 12.1.

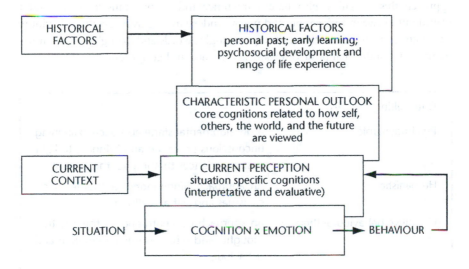

FIGURE 12.1   Integrated theoretical and applied model of stress and coping

Source: adapted from Katz and Hemmings (2009); reproduced with the permission of the British Psychological Society

This theoretical framework underpins interventions providing practitioners with a systematic understanding of athletes' presentations. This robust understanding is helpful to practitioners as it assists them with individual athlete case conceptualisations and intervention formulations.

This model is designed to be viewed as if it is three-dimensional, with the bottom level being most superficial and relating to what is being experienced in the current situation 'here and now'. This bottom level comprises environmental and psychological factors and the interactions between them. The psychological factors, represented within the rectangles, is further made up of cognitions and emotions and the interactions between them. The psychological factors are layered from current to historical psychological factors. Each layer has specific types of experience associated with it and the more general or global an athlete experiences something, the more important it is to them as a person, not 'just as an athlete'. Finally, each of the layers is located with the context in which that experience occurred.

It is sometimes argued that the theories and techniques of counselling are delivered through the presence and 'being' of the counsellor as a person (McLeod,

2011). No matter what the theoretical approach, much research suggests that the usefulness of the intervention of counselling comes from the quality of the relationship between client and practitioner (see, for example, Clarkson, 2007; Erskine, Moursund and Trautmann, 1999; McLeod, 2011; Moursund and Erskine, 2004). This relationship will usually convey trust and a deep sense of being special in the presence of another who demonstrates deep caring. Within an integrative approach, this is a safety felt where transference and countertransference are often played out between two people and where understanding over specific behaviours and emotions can be mediated through thought, words and 'being' in an environment of unconditional positive regard, acceptance and congruence.

Counselling models	
Psychodynamic	A developmental stage approach examining unconscious processes and bringing to light past experiences that impact the present.
Humanistic	An approach highlighting phenomenological issues and self-actualising.
Cognitive behavioural therapy	An approach concentrating on the way that thoughts and schemas impact emotion and behaviour.
Integrative	A theoretical approach examining the way that past and present collide in thought, emotion and behaviour.

Key skills

Each practitioner faces the challenge of translating their chosen therapeutic approach into practice. The application of theory into practice is achieved by the practitioner using a set of techniques or skills. The 'doing' of counselling, as opposed to the 'being' of counselling, can be seen as the skills used to build rapport and a strong working alliance with athletes. These attributes are represented in Figure 12.2. The main foundation skills recognised by practitioners of humanistic and integrative orientation are attending, observing, active listening, reflecting, probing, immediacy and challenge, all of which will be discussed below.

Attending skills

Attending skills refers to the set of skills the practitioner adopts to ensure an effective professional relationship. Attending acts as a basis for listening to and observing athletes; the means by which the practitioner communicates 'non-verbally' that they are 'with' their athlete and interested in them (Culley and Bond, 2007).

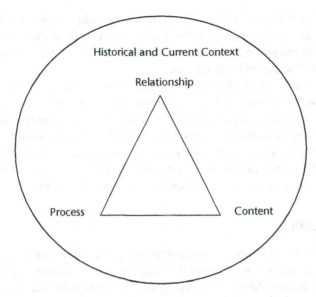

FIGURE 12.2 Overview of factors associated with the 1:1 consultation

Source: Katz & Hemmings (2009); reproduced with permission of the British Psychological Society.

Attending communicates acceptance and congruence. Attending and listening are inter-related; it is not possible to fully attend to athletes without listening to them. Attending to athletes allows verbal and non-verbal messages, and their contradictions between these verbal messages and behaviour, to be noticed (Egan, 2002). An open, upright and relaxed posture and good eye contact, without staring, are important (Culley and Bond, 2007).

Observing

Observing is the set of skills the practitioner uses to better understand the athlete's non-verbal behaviour and how this behaviour correlates, or not, with the athlete's verbal expression. Athletes communicate non-verbally through their dress, their tone of voice, facial expressions, gestures, postures, and so on, all of which inform the practitioner of inconsistencies between what athlete's verbalise and their behaviours. These observations offer opportunities for the practitioner and athlete to further explore inconsistencies for better understanding of presenting issues.

Active listening

Listening actively means listening with explicit purpose, using silences appropriately and communicating that you have listened and understood; it is about listening to, receiving and understanding messages whilst clarifying and organising information that is heard, checking what to respond to and asking for clarity on what is unclear (Culley and Bond, 2007). Active listening enables the practitioner to gain empathic understanding of the athlete's situation from their perspective. It provides useful insight into both what the athlete thinks and feels and the process of how these thoughts and feelings arise.

Using silences to further inform the process between practitioner and athlete is a necessary active listening skill that necessitates practitioners to be 'tuned in' to their athlete's emotional state. Listening to silences informs greatly about what is happening in the moment. Breaking silences should be for the client's benefit, used purposefully by the practitioner with a view to enhancing the therapeutic session, not to ease the practitioner's feelings of discomfort with silence or because of a lack of skill in working effectively with silence (Culley and Bond, 2007).

Reflective skills

The three reflective skills are restating, paraphrasing and summarising and these offer a way for the practitioner to construct how they communicate their empathic understanding (that is, from the athlete's perspective). Reflective skills help in the building of trust and empathy by offering to the athlete the practitioner's empathic understanding through active listening. This takes place with the professional relationship that provides 'time and space' within a safe environment and without imposing direction from the practitioner's frame of reference (Culley and Bond, 2007).

Restating involves repeating single key words or phrases back to the athlete to emphasise a point or an emotion. Paraphrasing lets the athlete know that the practitioner understands what they are saying by communicating back to them, in the practitioner's own words, the main message expressed by the athlete. Summarising organises the athlete's, sometimes disorganised, content by bringing together the salient aspects of their story (Culley and Bond, 2007). The consequence for athletes by practitioners using these skills is that they feel that they've been 'listened to' with their 'story' being valued, appreciated and understood.

Probing skills

Practitioners are sometimes required to question or gently challenge what athletes express and these are collectively referred to as 'probing skills'. 'We should use these skills with care; we may be going into areas where we haven't been invited' (Culley and Bond, 2007: 42). Probing offers opportunities for the client to explore issues that the practitioner thinks are important. The most helpful type of probing questions often begin with 'what, how, when, where and who' because they offer opportunity for open dialogue from the client rather than providing one-word responses.

Immediacy

Immediacy is a skill that involves listening to your own reactions as the practitioner and to use this to invite the athlete to look at what is happening between you and them. It is a very powerful tool because it invites immediate exploration of the athlete's feelings, thoughts and somatic responses. Using the skill of immediacy often feels risky for the practitioner because it involves verbalising a 'hunch' and, in so doing, inviting the client in to clarify what they are feeling or thinking in light of their immediate behaviour. Thus, it can be described as a coming together of the practitioner's feelings in the moment, and the athlete's behaviour in the moment, to make sense of what is going on in the relationship in that moment.

In much the same way as understanding transference and countertransference does within the psychodynamic approach, immediacy offers a way of interpreting what is going on in the therapeutic relationship. In relation to the humanistic approach, it is a way of focusing on the here and now of the practitioner and athlete. When relating it to a cognitive behavioural approach, it may be interpreted as using constructs to address patterns of relating between practitioner and athlete.

Of all the skills discussed, immediacy is a more advanced skill that tends to be used by more experienced practitioners, who will rely on their own highly tuned and acute self-awareness to provide valuable information to aid understanding of the client.

Fundamental counselling skills

- Attending skills.
- Observing clients.
- Active listening skills.
- Reflective skills (restating, paraphrasing, summarising).
- Probing skills (questioning).
- Immediacy.

A process of working

When injured, an athlete's physical injury is given primary attention, with the objective of providing diagnosis and subsequent medical and/or physical treatment. Thereafter, a process of recovery begins, which involves structured rehabilitation. This process is generally not linear but includes a variety of fluctuations associated with how the treatment and rehabilitation process meanders with ups and downs over time.

The continuous medical focus of the injury during treatment and rehabilitation can mask or hide underlying doubt and associated anxiety. Over time, and if this process is prolonged, the athlete can experience a disassociation between their medical care and how they feel psychologically about the impact and consequence of their injury. When anxiety expressed over an injury coincides with a pre-existing anxiety there may be a pattern of unhelpful behaviour that presents as challenging and confusing and that appears non-responsive to the more traditional mental skills work of sports psychology. As athletes' sense of identity is strongly associated with their sporting prowess, serious injury can be experienced as threatening to who they are as people and not just as athletes. Consequently, psychological recovery post-injury needs to support the athlete in re-establishing a sense of worth and value as a person before restoring their 'sporting confidence'.

Becoming injured can interrupt the usual physical and psychological homeostasis of the athlete. As discussed above, the physical aspects of the injury is the initial focus. Having identified potential long-term and significant psychological consequences to injury for some athletes, it is important to introduce psychological support as early in the process as is practical. Consequently, the earlier the practitioner can get involved within the treatment and rehabilitation process, the sooner the psychological and emotional needs of the athlete can be met, resulting in a more holistic process for the athlete. In this way, the person behind the athlete is also receiving support. This approach offers an environment within which the athlete can discuss the difficulties that their injury presents without fear of judgement and aside from the aspects of sporting performance within their rehabilitation. This type of psychological support places significance and importance of practitioner observation to ensure the practitioner is aware of the complete impact that the injury has had on the person behind the athlete and on their broader lifestyle. Further, good observation provides the opportunity for the practitioner to explore with athletes any potential secondary or underlying issues that may arise consequent to the physical injury.

Working with athletes requires a beginning, middle and an end to both the whole process and to each individual session. Typically, within the counselling relationship, the beginning of the whole process involves making an assessment, negotiating a contract, establishing boundaries, building trust and a working alliance, clarifying and defining difficult areas to explore together. The middle aspect of the process of counselling largely works to the contract negotiated at the beginning, maintains the working relationship and reassesses difficulties and concerns as they are worked through. Any end to the work, or part thereof, requires planning with mutual consent between practitioner and athlete. It is important to discuss the way in which this will occur, given that there may be consequences of ending the bond developed throughout working together. Thus, the process of emotional disengagement between practitioner and athlete requires respect within the work of 'ending' with an athlete. Some basic assumptions within this process are that people deserve acceptance and understanding, are capable of change, are experts on themselves, demonstrate behaviour that is purposeful and will work harder to achieve goals that are meaningful to them (Culley and Bond, 2007). Within all this, the individual, rather than their injury, is at the forefront of the work and this thereby allows for recognition of the athlete behind the injury.

An important aspect of working with clients is the recognition of attachment issues within the journey of eventual self-empowerment. Attachment can be seen as a bond between two people that involves a desire for regular contact with that person and experiencing discomfort when separated from that person (Ainsworth, 1989; Bowlby, 1979). An athlete's attachment style may present as dependency and some knowledge of how and when to gradually encourage them to regain control of their own choices about their treatment is a necessity for the aware practitioner.

Future directions

The role of the sport and exercise psychologist is changing (Aoyagi, Portenga, Poczwardowski, Cohen and Statler, 2012). Coaches are increasingly delivering mental skills training with their athletes, owing to developments in coach education. Increasingly, sports psychologists are supporting athletes who have concerns that have not been adequately or successfully managed through mental skills training alone. Thus, sports psychologists have a need for greater awareness of these issues within situations such as injury and rehabilitation. Working with peer support that allows space for discussion between practitioners about issues that may present in their athletes, is one way for the practitioner to reflect on their practice.

It must be stressed that any practitioner adopting such an approach should have a combination of high levels of self-awareness and the appropriate theoretical and applied training to be able to recognise the different aspects of the counselling 'process' that are inherent in an integrative theoretical underpinning and played out within the working alliance.

Conclusion

This chapter has highlighted a way of working with an athlete following injury that departs from the more traditional mental skills approach adopted to injury rehabilitation. The main aim of this chapter has been to offer an overview of theoretical approaches and skills to inform the practitioner when carrying out applied work with an injured athlete, and as such, it has suggested an alternative approach based on a counselling psychology model. To this end, the importance of 'the professional relationship' is paramount, since it bears the fruit of renewed hope for an athlete whose future has often been put in jeopardy through injury. This 'professional relationship', underpinned by an integrative theoretical approach within which specific skills can operate, is the framework within which practitioners might work should they be faced by an athlete who is either not responding to a mental skills approach or whose more complex range of underlying psychological issues requires a greater understanding through in-depth work.

CASE STUDY

Jill is a 15-year-old gymnast who injured her ankle during competition. She was referred to counselling by her sports psychologist, who recognised that Jill was presenting in a way that was posing a challenge for the sport psychologist and her physiotherapists, as she did not appear to recover as predicted. In essence, Jill's behaviour was making them feel as though they were out of their competency range; Jill was showing increasing amounts of erratic mood and resistance towards training and she appeared to present a tendency towards social avoidance. During the counselling sessions, Jill's eating behaviours and bodyweight issues came to light when Jill said 'it's hard to carry on in rhythmic gymnastics when girls start so young and are waif like. I used to be like that but once I got to fourteen, my body started to change and it was hard for me to eat the same things and keep my hips and legs slim'.

——————— **?** ———————

1. How might the models described in this chapter be used by different members of a multidisciplinary team?
2. When reading Jill's case study, how do you think counselling might help, over and above mental skills training?
3. Discuss what is meant by 'relationship'. Notice what emotions and physical feelings are evoked within you as you discuss this topic.

References

Ainsworth, M. (1989) Attachment beyond infancy. *American Psychologist*, 44, 709–16.
Aoyagi, M., Portenga, S., Poczwardowski, A., Cohen, A. and Statler, T. (2012) Reflections and directions: The profession of sport psychology past, present, and future. *Professional Psychology, Research and Practice*, 43(1), 32–38.
Beck, A. (1976) *Cognitive Therapy and the Emotional Disorders*. Harmondsworth: Penguin.
Bowlby, J. (1979) *The Making and Breaking of Affectional Bonds*. London: Tavistock.
Clarkson, P. (2007) *The Therapeutic Relationship*. London: Whurr.
Culley, S. and Bond, T. (2007) *Integrative Counselling Skills in Action*, 2nd edn. London: Sage.
Egan, G. (2002) *The Skilled Helper: A problem-management and opportunity-development approach to helping*, 7th edn. Pacific Grove, CA: Brooks/Cole.
Erskine, R., Moursund, J. and Trautmann, R. (1999) *Beyond Empathy: A therapy of contact-in-relationship*. London: Routledge.
Freud, S. (1949) *An Outline of Psychoanalysis*. London: Hogarth Press.
Gray, A. (2007) *An Introduction to the Therapeutic Frame*. London: Routledge.
Hough, M. (2006) *Counselling Skills and Theory*, 2nd edn. London: Hodder Arnold.
Jacobs, M. (1991) *Psychodynamic Counselling in Action*. London: Sage.
Katz, J. and Hemmings, B. (2009) *Counselling Skills Handbook for the Sport Psychologist*. Leicester: British Psychological Society.
Lapworth, P., Sills, C. and Fish, S. (2007) *Integration in Counselling and Psychotherapy: Developing a personal approach*. London: Sage.
McLeod, J. (2011) *An Introduction to Counselling*, 4th edn. Glasgow: McGraw Hill.
Moursund, J. P. and Erskine, R. G. (2004) *Integrative Psychotherapy: The art and science of relationship*. Pacific Grove, CA: Thomson: Brooks/Cole.
Rogers, C. (1963) The concept of the fully functioning person. *Psychotherapy: Theory, Research and Practice*, 1, 17–26.
Rogers, C. (1980) *A Way of Being*. Boston, MA: Houghton, Mifflin.
Wiese–Bjornstal, D. M., Smith, A. M., Shaffer, S. M. and Morrey, M. A. (1998) An integrated model of response to sport injury: Psychological and sociological dynamics. *Journal of Applied Sport Psychology*, 10, 46–69.

13

PSYCHOLOGY OF PHYSICAL ACTIVITY-RELATED INJURIES

Elaine A. Hargreaves and Julie A. Waumsley

Introduction

The physical and psychological benefits of participating in regular physical activity are well documented (see Powell, Paluch and Blair, 2011, for a review). Consequently, national health organisations and agencies (such as the World Health Organization; US Department of Health and Human Services, UK Department of Health) are directing health promotion efforts at encouraging the general population to engage in a physically active lifestyle. Current physical activity guidelines indicate that 150–300 minutes per week of moderate intensity activity (like walking) provides substantial health benefits, while similar benefits can also be achieved by 75 minutes per week of vigorous intensity activity or a combination of both moderate and vigorous intensity (Garber *et al.*, 2011; Powell *et al.*, 2011). Although the benefits of activity outweigh any risks, with the adoption of an active lifestyle or when the volume/intensity of activity being undertaken is increased suddenly (subsequently placing the individuals body under increased levels of stress) comes a greater exposure to the risk of injury (Andersen and Williams, 1988; Colbert, Hootman and Macera, 2000; Jones and Turner, 2005; Morrow, DeFina, Leonard, Trudelle-Jackson and Custodio, in press; Nicholl, Coleman and Williams, 1995).

Musculoskeletal injury is the most commonly reported adverse effect of physical activity (Hootman *et al.*, 2002; Janney and Jakicic, 2010; Powell *et al.*, 2011) and is frequently reported as the reason for ceasing involvement in activity (Hootman *et al.*, 2002; Sallis *et al.*, 1990) or as a barrier to increasing physical activity (Finch, Owen and Price, 2001; Toscos, Consolvo and McDonald, 2011). Additionally, simply having a fear of injury has been reported as a major barrier to the adoption of an active lifestyle (Booth, Bauman, Owen and Gore, 1997; Eyler, Brownson, Bacak and Housemann, 2003).

Consequently, it is surprising that, thus far, very little research has focused on the response to injury in a recreationally active population. Research related to the psychological responses to injury has predominately focused on recreational sport and competitive athletes (see Walker, Thatcher and Lavallee, 2007; Wiese-Bjornstal, 2010, for reviews of this literature; Wiese-Bjornstal, Smith, Shaffer and Morrey, 1998) or on clinical populations (for example, chronic low back pain, Vlaeyen, Kole-Snijders, Boeren and van Eek, 1995). Given the direct impediment to physical activity participation that results from injury (or simply having fear of injury) and the likely adverse effect on motivation for activity following an injury in this population, a discussion of these issues is warranted.

This chapter discusses the existing research on the psychological responses to injury in recreationally active populations and draws from sport injury response models to study the psychology of activity-related injury. More specifically, the chapter: a) discusses injury prevalence from physical activity; b) identifies the psychological consequences associated with physical activity related injuries; c) applies the integrated model of psychological response to the sport injury and rehabilitation process (Wiese-Bjornstal, *et al.*, 1998) into the physical activity injury context; d) examines the existing literature on the appraisal processes and emotional and behavioural responses to physical activity-related injuries; and e) introduces psychological interventions that can be used when recovering from physical activity related injuries.

Physical activity-related injuries: prevalence

Reporting the prevalence of activity-related injuries is not straightforward because reports typically combine sport and physical activity-related injuries together in one category and the method used to report prevalence differs (see, for example, Burt and Overpeck, 2001; Carlson *et al.*, 2006; Uitenbroek, 1996). Studies which have reported injury prevalence in physically active and sedentary individuals show that the type and intensity of physical activity are important considerations (Garber *et al.*, 2011). Walking and moderate-intensity activity are associated with lower risk of injury compared with jogging/running and more vigorous intensity activities (Table 13.1).

Despite a perception by exercisers that participation in physical activity is not associated with a high risk of injury (Finch, Otago, White, Donaldson and Mahoney, 2011), these statistics would suggest that injuries resulting from physical activity are just as prevalent as those that result from sport. Risk factors for injury in a physically active population include engaging in more than 1.25 hours of activity per week (Hootman *et al.*, 2001), having a higher level of fitness (Colbert, Hootman and Macera, 2000; Hootman *et al.*, 2002; Hootman *et al.*, 2001), having had a previous injury (Colbert *et al.*, 2000; Hootman *et al.*, 2002; Morrow, DeFina, Leonard, Trudelle-Jackson and Custodio, 2012; Requa, DeAvilla and Garrick, 1993) and having a higher body mass index (Janney and Jakicic, 2010). When injury statistics are adjusted for actual physical activity exposure time, there is an increased risk of injury and prolonged healing time with increasing age (Finch *et al.*, 2001).

TABLE 13.1 Injury prevalence from common physical activities

Type of physical activity	Intensity	Prevalence (%) Men	Women	Reference
Walking	Moderate	7–17	18–20	Colbert et al., (2000); Hootman et al., (2002; 2001)
Jogging/running	Vigorous	25–64	23–44	Colbert et al., (2000); Hootman et al., (2002; 2001)
Gardening; DIY; cycling	Moderate	Relatively low, but high participation rates = higher injury rates		Powell et al., (1998), Parkkari et al., (2004)
Fitness activities: running, weight training and keep fit	Moderate to vigorous	> 2 million exercise-related incidents annually in the UK 49.6	33.8	Nicholl et al., (1995); Lubetzky-Vilnai et al. (2009)

As more individuals answer the call by national health organisations and agencies to participate in physical activity, and with a high proportion of those individuals likely to be at risk of injury (for example, older in age, overweight), it is likely that the prevalence of injuries will increase (Green and Weinberg, 2001; Parkkari et al., 2004).

Physical activity related injuries: consequences

Finch, Owen and Price (2001) highlighted the myriad adverse outcomes that can be experienced as the result of a physical activity-related injury. Similarly to athletic injuries, an individual's overall health can be affected through physical and psychological impairment. On occasions, there can be financial implications if the injury influences the individual's ability to work. For the majority of individuals, an activity-related injury results in a temporary cessation or reduction of physical activity levels but for some it can put a more permanent stop to their activity levels, despite the injury only being a temporary impairment (Hootman et al., 2002; Janney and Jakicic, 2010; Powell, Heath, Kresnow, Sacks and Branche, 1998; Sallis et al., 1990). Furthermore, only 25 per cent experiencing an activity-related injury seek treatment (Nicholl, Coleman and Williams, 1995; although this number was greater in those who meet the physical activity guidelines, Morrow et al., 2012; Powell et al., 1998) and only 30–40 per cent perform rehabilitation exercises (Hootman et al., 2002). Thus, the risk of future injury is increased, owing to the lack of proper injury treatment and rehabilitation. More importantly, perhaps, owing to the reduction or permanent cessation of physical activity behaviour, individuals will no longer be able to gain the widespread physiological and psychological health benefits of an active lifestyle. Therefore, if an injury occurs the main concerns are to ensure individuals rehabilitate properly and return to a phys-ically active lifestyle.

Sallis *et al.* (1990) showed that some individuals will return to activity follow-ing an injury related relapse and others will not, suggesting that there are some underlying psychological mechanisms that explain post-injury activity behaviour. The study of psychological responses to injury in the sport context has drawn mainly from cognitive appraisal and stress process frameworks (see, for example, Wiese-Bjornstal, 2010; Wiese-Bjornstal, Smith and LaMott, 1995; Wiese-Bjornstal *et al.*, 1998; see also Chapter 3). In the physical activity context, whether or not an individual returns to their pre-injury physical activity patterns and/or adheres to any necessary injury rehabilitation will be influenced by his or her cognitive appraisal of, and affective reactions to, their injury. These behavioural attempts then have their own set of consequences (for example, success, experience of pain) that will feed back into the cognitive and affective appraisal process (Wiese-Bjornstal, 2010). Although there is limited direct research to support the proposals of the framework in an activity-related injury context, indirect support can be drawn from sport and general injury contexts, as well as related research from the psychol-ogy of physical activity.

Physical activity-related injuries: an integrated model of psychological response to the sport injury and rehabilitation process (Wiese-Bjornstal *et al.*, 1998)

Discrete aspects of the consequences to injury resulting from physical activity are difficult to tease apart. The cognitive appraisals of the initial injury followed by the emotional and behavioural responses that result, interact and, additionally, are moderated by personal and situational factors. This is illustrated in the following discussion and in the case study at the end of the chapter.

Goals

For those individuals who are trying to become regularly active, physical activity is typically a goal-directed behaviour (Sebire, Standage and Vansteenkiste, 2009). The nature of, and reasons for, the goal achievement influence psychological outcomes (Sebire *et al.*, 2009) and thereby the cognitive appraisal of an injury. For those moti-vated to achieve tangible rewards from their activity, such as enhanced appearance, the occurrence of an injury will suspend the achievement of those goals. Perceptions of not making progress towards achieving goals produces distressing emotional states and disrupts self-regulation of behaviour (Berger, Pargman and Weinberg, 2006; Maddux and Gosselin, 2003). This extrinsic form of motivation is more prevalent in individuals who are in the early stages of physical activity behav-iour change (Wilson, Mack and Grattan, 2008) and this appraisal will put them at risk of ceasing their involvement in physical activity.

In comparison, for individuals who are regularly active, motivation for physical activity often comes from a sense of enjoyment and because it is a valued behaviour (Wilson *et al.*, 2008). For these individuals, the occurrence of an injury may carry a great sense of loss. From a cognitive appraisal perspective individuals who have higher commitment to physical activity will experience greater negative emotional responses including, guilt, depression, irritability, restlessness, tension, stress, anxiety and sluggishness because the injury prevents them from being active (Chan and Grossman, 1988; Green and Weinberg, 2001; Hausenblas and Symons Downs, 2002; Johnston and Carroll, 2000b). Despite having a negative affective response to forced inactivity, it is likely that regularly active individuals will take the steps necessary to return to their pre-injury activity levels and will adhere to treatment because of the value and positive benefits they experience from being active (King-Chung Chan, Hagger and Spray, 2011; Levy, Polman, Nicholls and Marchant, 2009).

Identity

An individual's self-identity can be encapsulated within their role as an exerciser (Strachan, Flora, Brawley and Spink, 2011). With injury comes an inability to fulfil this role, resulting in a challenge to this identity which can lead to cognitive and affective reactions (Collinson and Hockey, 2007; Strachan *et al.*, 2011; Wiese-Bjornstal, 2004). Strachan *et al.* (2011) found that, with a strong exercise identity, being unable to exercise led to a negative affective response, which they suggested acts as a motivator to return to activity so as to regain consistency between identity and behaviour. Research in the sport context has shown that with a particularly severe injury or if recovery is slower than hoped, then athletic identity decreases over time (Brewer, Cornelius, Stephan and Van Raalte, 2010). This decrease is suggested to protect self-concept and reduce the experience of negative affect because the individual devalues that aspect of themselves to reduce the discrepancy between identity (for example, 'I am an exerciser') and actual behaviour (for example, 'I am not exercising'). However, this change in identity may compromise the return to activity.

Self-efficacy

Self-efficacy is an individual's belief in his or her abilities (Bandura, 1997). Self-efficacy is one of the strongest determinants of participation in physical activity and influences affective and cognitive outcomes of physical activity (Biddle and Mutrie, 2008; Trost, France and Thomas, 2011). Consequently, following an injury, the individual's appraisal of their self-efficacy will be prominent in the psychological response to injury and will influence future behaviour, including adherence to rehabilitation. There are a variety of self-efficacy beliefs that operate in the physical activity domain. Task self-efficacy refers to the individual's ability to complete certain activities (for example, walk for 30 minutes, perform strength training exercises). The period of inactivity caused by the injury is likely to reduce perceptions of task self-efficacy such that the individual will not feel as able to perform activities to the same level after the injury as they did before injury. Importantly, task self-efficacy is negatively associated with a fear of re-injury (Tripp, Stanish, Ebel-Lam, Brewer and Birchard, 2007). Barrier self-efficacy refers to the individual's ability to overcome environmental and personal barriers that exist to being active. With an injury comes new barriers to negotiate (such as changing to another form of activity). Recovery self-efficacy (an ability to resume a behaviour after a lapse) also influences future activity levels (Luszczynska, Mazurkiewicz, Ziegelmann and Schwarzer, 2007) and adherence to rehabilitation (Levy, Polman and Clough, 2008). The individual's ability to maintain and/or build their self-efficacy following injury will influence the likelihood of returning to regular activity and adhering to rehabilitation.

It's been brilliant to work with a specialist in exercise psychology through my injury. I didn't actually know they existed, or what they did, and I was a bit sceptical at first! But speaking with Lisa has helped me recognise the negative thought patterns I have had since my injury and how they have contributed to me feeling frustrated, moody and lacking motivation for rehab. I felt so overwhelmed with all the exercises the physio gave me and they were so painful to begin with that I did everything possible to avoid doing them. I couldn't see I would ever get back to my old running routine.

But with Lisa I set some achievable goals for doing my exercises, we worked on changing my negative thoughts about the pain into positive ones so I could cope with the pain better and she got me to realise that getting injured wasn't the end of the world. I think the sense of control I got back from a situation that I didn't really feel in control of really helped. I have learned so much about myself and now much better understand why I react to things the way I do and what the consequences are. It's still hard work and I still catch myself following old patterns, but I can now recognise when I go into a slump and I can give myself a good talking too! So it's been worth it really, if I hadn't spoken to a specialist in exercise psychology and got her support I probably wouldn't have stuck with the rehab and got back to being active.

(John, recreational runner)

Causal attributions

Physical activity-related injuries can result from a number of situations and can activate thoughts related to the cause of the injury which will influence the affective and behavioural response (Wiese-Bjornstal, 2004). The cause of injury can be attributed to internal or external (personal/environmental) factors, can be stable or unstable (unchangeable/ changeable) and can be perceived as personally controllable or not. Extrapolating findings in sport to the context of activity–injury suggests that if the individual takes personal responsibility for the injury, perceives that the causal factors do not change over time but are personally controllable then an adaptive psychological and behavioural response will result (Brewer, 1999; Coffee and Rees, 2009; Shields, Brawley and Lindover, 2005).

Coping skills

The extent to which the individual feels they have appropriate coping resources and skills is proposed to influence their cognitive appraisal of the injury (Wiese-Bjornstal *et al.*, 1998). Additionally, the extent to which the individual implements strategies to manage the stress presented by the injury is suggested as a behavioural outcome of the stress appraisal process (Wiese-Bjornstal, 2010). Coping skills are typically defined according to two main processes: problem-focused coping, which refers to cognitive and behavioural attempts to manage or change the problem that is causing the stress (for example, accepting the injury and focusing on rehabilitation) and emotion-focused coping, which refers to attempts to regulate the emotional response to the problem (for example, expressing negative emotions; Lazarus and Folkman, 1984). Research would suggest that problem-focused coping strategies are more advantageous compared with emotion-focused coping (Johnston and Carroll, 2000a; Quinn and Fallon, 1999). For a review of common coping strategies employed in medical situations, see Wiese-Bjornstal (2004).

Social support

Social support is a key situational factor that can influence the psychological response to physical activity related injury in a number of ways. In the initial cognitive appraisal, it can reduce the perceptions of stress posed by the injury (Uchino, 2009), improve affective reactions (Rees, Mitchell, Evans and Hardy, 2010) and build self-efficacy (Podlog and Eklund, 2007). The nature and provider of the social support is important (Collinson and Hockey, 2007; DiMatteo, 2004; Podlog and Eklund, 2007; Uchino, 2009). Sport medicine professionals will likely provide informational support, while family and friends will likely provide emotional support and, if the injury is severe, will provide practical support (for more details on providers of social support, see Chapter 9). Importantly, with a physical activity-related injury comes the potential loss of support provided by those who the individual regularly exercises with and the possibility to feel socially isolated (Podlog and Eklund, 2007). Thus, the individual's ability to mobilise appropriate social support from other sources will influence their appraisal of their injury. Uchino (2009) explains that the effects of social support are not always positive, particularly if it reduces the individuals sense of independence or if the provider of social support does not provide the right kind of support.

A response to physical activity-related injuries typically follows a pattern of:

- cognitive appraisal (e.g. goal adjustment; self-perceptions);
- emotional responses (e.g. re-injury anxiety; loss);
- behavioural responses (e.g. activity continuation; adherence to rehabilitation);
- in response to the injury, an exerciser's cognitive appraisals, emotional and behavioural responses interact (known as the dynamic core);
- the dynamic core responses are all moderated by personal (e.g., activity experience) and situational (e.g. social support) factors;
- the dynamic core will have an impact on the overall physical and psychological recovery, and vice versa.

Pain perceptions and fear of re-injury/re-injury anxiety

Injuries can often result in pain. Individuals who engage in catastrophising focus excessively on pain sensations (rumination), exaggerate the threat of pain sensations (magnification) and doubt their ability to cope effectively with situations that induce pain (helplessness) (Sullivan, Bishop and Pivik, 1995). The extent to which individuals engage in catastrophising may influence the intensity of pain experienced as a result of injury, influence adherence to injury rehabilitation exercises (particularly if they result in some pain) and may influence confidence in being able to return to physical activity. Fear of injury, and/or re-injury anxiety are a common response in those who return to sport following an injury and these can be a major barrier to participation in physical activity (e.g., Finch *et al.*, 2001; Toscos *et al.*, 2011). The experience of pain from the initial injury contributes to fears and/or anxieties about re-injury because the individual is worried that they will suffer further pain (Sullivan *et al.*, 2002). It is useful here to recognise that 'fear' and 're-injury anxiety' are two separate concepts, yet they might be experienced independently or concurrently during rehabilitation and return to training and competition (Walker and Thatcher, 2011).

Suggested psychological interventions for rehabilitation and resuming physical activity

The following practical strategies are based on the previous discussion and sports injury literature, which suggests that, to help individuals overcome their activity-related injury, the focus should be to reduce the threat appraisal presented by the injury (Levy *et al.*, 2008). The rationale being:

1. It will enable a more positive psychological response to the injury.
2. It will enable the individual to feel more optimistic about recovery.
3. It will enable a return to pre-injury levels of activity.

Key strategies for promoting adherence to injury rehabilitation and the resumption of physical activity

Goal setting:
- Suspend previous activity-related goals while injured to reduce the sense of non-accomplishment of goals and create new 'achievable' goals for the rehabilitation period.
- Replace old physical activity routines with a new rehabilitation routine.
- On return to activity, new activity goals should acknowledge the individuals lowered level of functioning post-injury to limit the risk of re-injury and build self-efficacy.
- Recognise the enjoyment and value gained from being active and not just the extrinsic rewards.

Imagery:
- Imagine successfully performing rehabilitation exercises.
- Imagine being active without pain.
- Imagine being active at pre-injury capabilities.

Positive self-talk:
- Reframe negative thoughts.
- Celebrate successes; give positive feedback.

Personal control:
- Identify how to overcome new barriers to activity presented by injury.
- Take responsibility for the occurrence of injury and the rehabilitation.

Social support:
- Seek out appropriate social support from general practitioners, physiotherapists, family and friends to provide emotional and practical support.
- Connect with activity friends in other ways (for example, attend the after activity social occasion).

Self-identity:
- Maintain pre-injury habits where possible (for example, wear exercise attire during rehabilitation, use the same activity locations during recovery).
- Recognise other aspects of life that bring meaning and enjoyment.
- Maintain identity as an exerciser. The break is only temporary.

Conclusion

This chapter has discussed research on psychological responses to injury in recreationally active populations and has used sport injury response models and other health behaviour theories to study the psychology of activity-related injury. Drawing from a cognitive appraisal and stress framework and injury research from sport and clinical populations, this chapter has highlighted the interactions that exist between the cognitive appraisal of the initial injury and the resulting emotional and behavioural responses, as well as the role that personal and situational factors play in moderating those responses. Owing to the lack of direct research on the topic, it is by no means an exhaustive account and other factors identified as important to the psychological outcomes of sport injury (for example, personality factors; Wiese-Bjornstal, 2010; Wiese-Bjornstal et al., 1998) have not been discussed but may be important to the appraisal of an activity-related injury. Furthermore, most of the outcomes proposed throughout have still to be confirmed through experimental research and would make for an exciting programme of research.

CASE STUDY

Amanda is a 33-year-old white female who, after being relatively inactive for the last five years (*personal factor*), has been attending a weekly 'spinning' class for the last month. She goes for several reasons (*goals*): she wants to lose a bit of weight and to feel fitter and mentally healthier. She has recognised that she feels more 'upbeat' when she's active and because she meets her friends at the class, she enjoys it as a social occasion. When Amanda suffered a calf injury, it became too painful for her to cycle and she had to rest. As a consequence, she gained weight, she felt less healthy and she missed out on socialising with her friends. The forced rest from the injury meant that she could not achieve her goals (*cognitive appraisal*) and this resulted in her feeling frustrated, irritable and a little 'down' (*emotional response*). She also missed the motivational support she got from her friends (*situational factor*). As time drifted on, Amanda's motivation to return to the class waned because she no longer saw the point in being active, wasn't getting any emotional or practical support and she was worried that she would just get injured again.

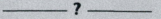 **?**

1. What do you consider to be the most important aspects that an exercise psychology specialist should consider when working with a recreationally active individual with an injury?
2. If putting together a psychological programme of rehabilitation for a recreationally active individual with an injury, what would you consider?
3. How do you see Wiese-Bjornstal's (2010) model contributing to activity-related injury?

References

Andersen, M. B. and Williams, J. M. (1988) A model of stress and athletic injury: Prediction and prevention. *Journal of Sport and Exercise Psychology*, 10, 294–306.

Bandura, A. (1997) *Self-efficacy: The exercise of control.* New York: Freeman.

Berger, B. G., Pargman, D. and Weinberg, R. S. (eds) (2006) *Factors Influencing Exercise-related Injury and Factors Related to Rehabilitation Adherence*, 3rd edn. Morgantown, WV: Fitness Information Technology.

Biddle, S., J H and Mutrie, N. (2008) *Psychology of Physical Activity: Determinants, well-being and interventions*, 2nd edn. London: Routledge.

Booth, M. L., Bauman, A., Owen, N. and Gore, C. J. (1997) Physical activity preferences, preferred sources of assistance, and perceived barriers to increased activity among physically inactive Australians. *Preventive Medicine*, 26, 131–7.

Brewer, B. W. (1999) Causal attribution dimensions and adjustment to sport injury. *Journal of Personal and Interpersonal Loss*, 4, 215–24.

Brewer, B. W., Cornelius, A. E., Stephan, Y. and Van Raalte, J. (2010) Self-protective changes in athletic identity following anterior cruciate ligament reconstruction. *Psychology of Sport and Exercise*, 11, 1–5.

Burt, C. W. and Overpeck, M. D. (2001) Emergency visits for sports-related injuries. *Annals of Emergency Medicine*, 37(3), 301–8.

Carlson, S. A., Hootman, J. M., Powell, K. E., Macera, C. A., Heath, G. W., Gilchrist, J. and Kohl, H. W. I. (2006) Self-reported injury and physical activity levels: United States 2000–2002. *Annuals of Epidemiology*, 16, 712–9.

Chan, C. S. and Grossman, H. Y. (1988) Psychological effects of running loss on consistent runners. *Perceptual and Motor Skills*, 66, 875–83.

Coffee, P. and Rees, T. (2009) The main and interactive effects of immediate and reflective attributions upon subsequent self-efficacy. *European Journal of Sport Sciences*, 9(1), 41–52.

Colbert, L. H., Hootman, J. M. and Macera, C. A. (2000) Physical activity-related injuries in walkers and runners in the aerobics center longitudinal study. *Clinical Journal of Sport Medicine*, 10, 259–63.

Collinson, J. A. and Hockey, J. (2007) 'Working out' identity: Distance runners and the management of disrupted identity. *Leisure Studies*, 26(4), 381–98.

DiMatteo, M. R. (2004) Social support and patient adherence to medical treatment: A meta-analysis. *Health Psychology*, 23(2), 207–18.

Eyler, A. A., Brownson, R. C., Bacak, S. J. and Housemann, R. A. (2003) The epidemiology of walking for physical activity in the United States. *Medicine and Science in Sports and Exercise*, 35(9), 1529–36.

Finch, C. F., Otago, L., White, P., Donaldson, A. and Mahoney, M. (2011) The safety attitudes of people who use multi-purpose recreation facilities as a physical activity setting. *International Journal of Injury, Control and Safety Promotion*, 18(2), 107–12.

Finch, C. F., Owen, N. and Price, R. (2001) Current injury or disability as a barrier to being more physically active. *Medicine and Science in Sports and Exercise*, 33, 778–82.

Garber, C. E., Blissmer, B., Deschenes, M. R., Franklin, B. A., Lamonte, M. J., Lee, I. and Swain, D. P. (2011) Quantity and quality of exercise for developing and maintaining cardiorespiratory, musculoskeletal, and neuromotor fitness in apparently health adults: Guidance for prescribing exercise. *Medicine and Science in Sports and Exercise*, 43(7), 1334–1359. doi: 10.1249/MSS.0b013e318213fefb.

Green, S. L. and Weinberg, R. S. (2001) Relationships among athletic identity, coping skills, social support, and the psychological impact of injury in recreational participants. *Journal of Applied Sport Psychology*, 13(1), 40–59.

Hausenblas, H. A. and Symons Downs, D. (2002) Exercise dependence: A systematic review. *Psychology of Sport and Exercise*, 3, 89–123.

Hootman, J. M., Macera, C. A., Ainsworth, B. E., Addy, C. L., Martin, M. and Blair, S. N. (2002) Epidemiology of musculoskeletal injuries among sedentary and physically active individuals. *Medicine and Science in Sports and Exercise*, 34(5), 838–44.

Hootman, J. M., Macera, C. A., Ainsworth, B. E., Martin, M., Addy, C. L. and Blair, S. N. (2001) Association among physical activity level, cardiorespiratory fitness, and risk of musculoskeletal injury. *American Journal of Epidemiology*, 154(3), 251–258.

Janney, C. A. and Jakicic, J. M. (2010) The influence of exercise and BMI on injuries and illnesses in overweight and obese individuals: A randomized control trial. *International Journal of Behavioral Nutrition and Physical Activity*, 7(1). doi: 10.1186/1479-5868-7-1.

Johnston, L. H. and Carroll, D. (2000a) Coping, social support, and injury: Changes over time and the effects of level of sports involvement. *Journal of Sport Rehabilitation*, 9, 290–303.

Johnston, L. H. and Carroll, D. (2000b) The psychological impact of injury: Effects of prior sport and exercise involvement. *British Journal of Sports Medicine*, 34, 436–9.

Jones, C. S. and Turner, L. W. (2005) Non-equipment exercise-related injuries among U.S. women 65 and older: Emergency department visits from 1994–2001. *Journal of Women and Aging*, 17, 71–81.

King-Chung Chan, D., Hagger, M. S. and Spray, C. M. (2011) Treatment motivation for rehabilitation after a sport injury: Application of the trans-contextual model. *Psychology of Sport & Exercise*, 12, 83–92.

Lazarus, R. and Folkman, S. (1984) *Stress, Appraisal and Coping.* New York: Springer.

Levy, A. R., Polman, R. C. J. and Clough, P. J. (2008) Adherence to sport injury rehabilitation programs: An integrated psycho-social approach. *Scandinavian Journal of Medicine and Science in Sports*, 18, 798–809.

Levy, A. R., Polman, R. C. J., Nicholls, A. R. and Marchant, D. C. (2009) Sport injury rehabilitation adherence: Perspectives of recreational athletes. *International Journal of Sport and Exercise Psychology*, 7(2), 212–29.

Luszczynska, A., Mazurkiewicz, M., Ziegelmann, J. P. and Schwarzer, R. (2007) Recovery self-efficacy and intention as predictors of running or jogging behavior: A cross-lagged panel analysis over a two-year period. *Psychology of Sport and Exercise*, 8, 247–60.

Maddux, J. E. and Gosselin, J. T. (2003) Self-efficacy. In M. R. Leary and J. Price (eds), *Handbook of Self and Identity.* New York: Guilford Press, pp. 218–38.

Morrow, J. R., DeFina, L. F., Leonard, D., Trudelle-Jackson, E. and Custodio, M. A. (2012) Meeting physical activity guidelines and musculoskeletal injury: The WIN study. *Medicine and Science in Sports and Exercise*, 44(10), 1986–92.

Nicholl, J. P., Coleman, P. and Williams, B. T. (1995) The epidemiology of sports and exercise related injury in the United Kingdom. *British Journal of Sports Medicine*, 29(4), 232–38.

Parkkari, J., Kannus, P., Natri, A., Lapinleimu, I., Palvanen, M., Heiskanen, M., and Järvinen, M. (2004) Active living and injury risk. *International Journal of Sports Medicine*, 25, 209–16.

Podlog, L. and Eklund, R. C. (2007) The psychosocial aspects of a return to sport following serious injury: A review of the literature from a self-determination theory perspective. *Psychology of Sport and Exercise*, 8, 535–66.

Powell, K. E., Heath, G. W., Kresnow, M., Sacks, J. J. and Branche, C. M. (1998) Injury rates from walking, gardening, weightlifting, outdoor bicycling, and aerobics. *Medicine and Science in Sports and Exercise*, 30(8), 1246–9.

Powell, K. E., Paluch, A. E. and Blair, S. N. (2011) Physical activity for health: What kind? How much? How intense? On top of what? *Annual Review of Public Health*, 32(3), 349–65.

Quinn, A. M. and Fallon, B. J. (1999) The changes in psychological characteristics and reactions of elite athletes from injury onset until full recovery. *Journal of Applied Sport Psychology*, 11, 210–29.

Rees, T., Mitchell, I., Evans, L. and Hardy, L. (2010) Stressors, social support and psychological reactions to sport injury in high- and low-performance standard participants. *Psychology of Sport and Exercise*, 11, 505–12.

Requa, R. K., DeAvilla, L. N. and Garrick, J. G. (1993) Injuries in recreational adult fitness activities. *American Journal of Sports Medicine*, 21(3), 461–7.

Sallis, J. F., Hovell, M. F., Hofstetter, C. R., Elder, J. P., Faucher, P., Spry, V. M., and Hackley, M. (1990) Lifetime history of relapse from exercise. *Addictive Behaviors*, 15, 573–9.

Sebire, S. J., Standage, M. and Vansteenkiste, M. (2009) Examining intrinsic versus extrinsic exercise goals: Cognitive, affective, and behavioural outcomes. *Journal of Sport and Exercise Psychology*, 31, 189–210.

Shields, C. A., Brawley, L. R. and Lindover, T. I. (2005) Where perception and reality differ: Dropping out is not the same as failure. *Journal of Behavioral Medicine*, 25(5), 481–91.

Strachan, S. M., Flora, P. K., Brawley, L. R. and Spink, K. S. (2011) Varying the cause of a challenge to exercise identity behaviour: Reactions of individuals of differing identity strength. *Journal of Health Psychology*, 16(4), 572–83.

Sullivan, M. J. L., Bishop, S. and Pivik, J. (1995) The pain catastrophizing scale: Development and validation. *Psychological Assessment*, 7, 524–32.

Sullivan, M. J. L., Rodgers, W. M., Wilson, P. M., Bell, G. J., Murray, T. C. and Fraser, S. N. (2002) An experimental investigation of the relation between catastrophizing and activity intolerance. *Pain*, 100, 47–53.

Toscos, T., Consolvo, S. and McDonald, D. W. (2011) Barriers to physical activity: A study of self-revelation in an online community. *Journal of Medical Systems*, 35(5), 1225–42. doi: 10.1007/s10916–011–9721–2.

Tripp, D. A., Stanish, W., Ebel–Lam, A., Brewer, B. W. and Birchard, J. (2007) Fear of reinjury, negative affect, and catastrophizing predicting return to sport in recreational athletes with anterior cruciate ligament injuries at 1 year postsurgery. *Rehabilitation Psychology*, 52(1), 74–81.

Trost, Z., France, C. R. and Thomas, J. S. (2011) Pain-related fear and avoidance of physical exertion following delayed-onset muscle soreness. *Pain*, 152(7), 1540–7.

Uchino, B. N. (2009) Understanding the links between social support and physical health: A lifespan perspective with emphasis on the separability of perceived and received support. *Perspectives on Psychological Science*, 4(3), 236–55.

Uitenbroek, D. G. (1996) Sports, exercise, and other causes of injuries: Results of a population survey. *Research Quarterly for Exercise and Sport*, 67(4), 380–5.

Vlaeyen, J. W. S., Kole-Snijders, A. M. J., Boeren, R. G. B. and van Eek, H. (1995) Fear of movement/(re)injury in chronic low back pain and its relation to behavioural performance. *Pain*, 62, 363–72.

Walker, N. and Thatcher, J. (2011) The emotional response to athletic injury: Re–injury anxiety. In J. Thatcher, M. Jones and D. Lavallee (eds), *Coping and Emotion in Sport*, 2nd edn. New York: Routledge, pp. 236–60.

Walker, N., Thatcher, J. and Lavallee, D. (2007) Psychological responses to injury in competitive sport: A critical review. *Journal of the Royal Society for the Promotion of Health*, 127(4), 174–80.

Wiese-Bjornstal, D. M. (2004) Psychological responses to injury and illness. In G. S. Kolt and M. B. Andersen (eds), *Psychology in the Physical and Manual Therapies*. Edinburgh: Churchill Livingstone, pp. 21–38.

Wiese-Bjornstal, D. M. (2010) Psychology and socioculture affect injury risk, response, and recovery in high-intensity athletes: a consensus statement. *Scandinavian Journal of Medicine and Science in Sports*, 20, 103–11.

Wiese-Bjornstal, D. M., Smith, A. M. and LaMott, E. E. (1995) A model of psychologic response to athletic injury and rehabilitation. *Athletic Training: Sports Health Care Perspectives*, 1(1), 17–30.

Wiese-Bjornstal, D. M., Smith, A. M., Shaffer, S. M. and Morrey, M. A. (1998) An integrated model of responses to sport injury: Psychological and sociological dynamics. *Journal of Applied Sport Psychology*, 10, 46–69.

Wilson, P. M., Mack, D. E. and Grattan, K. P. (2008) Understanding motivation for exercise: A self-determination theory perspective. *Canadian Psychology*, 49(3), 250–6.

14

CONCLUSIONS AND FUTURE DIRECTIONS

Natalie Walker and Monna Arvinen-Barrow

It has been the aim of this book to demonstrate the ways in which psychology can play a role in the sport injury process. Moreover, the book has aimed to provide the reader with a comprehensive view of the subject matter by adopting a holistic perspective incorporating theory, research and applied knowledge when discussing the usefulness of psychological interventions and counselling skills in sport injury rehabilitation. By doing so, the text has also demonstrated how much the subject area involving psychology of sport injuries has advanced since the early 1990s, at which time several text books focusing on this topic emerged. Collectively, the three parts within the current text draw on some of the early work and present an outline of the more diverse and established literature and practitioner suggestions, thus allowing a provision of evidence-based suggestions for sport medicine practitioners, athletes, and researchers.

In Part 1, Chapter 1 highlighted the importance of addressing psychological issues during rehabilitation to ensure a full and holistic recovery. The subsequent chapters then introduced the key terminology and relevant theories and models. The models outlined provided useful frameworks that can be used by those interacting with injured athletes and help them to understand the athletes' experiences and the potential impact of such experiences on the individual – from injury onset to full recovery. Chapter 2 introduced the stress and injury model and, although it was introduced over 20 years ago, this model still remains the single most dominant framework in guiding researchers today in the prediction and prevention of sport injury. With this in mind, those working in the applied setting should consider educating athletes about the importance of good health and adopting a healthy lifestyle for minimising the risk of injury. Moreover, coaches and sport medicine professionals alike should get to know their athletes, should be sensitive to any increased stress levels and should subsequently assist them in using relevant skills and techniques to help manage their cognitive appraisals, emotions, and behaviours.

As demonstrated in Chapter 3, the importance of theoretical frameworks should not be limited to injury onset but should extend to psychological responses to injury, the impact of these responses on rehabilitation and subsequent return to sport. Whilst much of the early work on responses to injury was adopted from the grief domain, and subsequently heavily criticised, it would still be advantageous to explore the usefulness of more contemporary grief models as a framework in this area. Researchers are encouraged to continue to use the cognitive appraisal and biopsychosocial models as frameworks for exploring the athlete's responses to sport injury and to generate more information to help guide sport medicine profession-als in addressing adverse psychological responses to injuries and enhancing adherence to rehabilitation. The latter is vitally important, as highlighted in Chapter 4, the significance of rehabilitation adherence as an essential component for success-ful rehabilitation cannot be doubted. It is also evident that non-adherence is associated with poor rehabilitation outcomes and increases the risk of re-injury. Thus, applied practitioners are encouraged to create an environment that is conducive to adherence (see Chapters 11 and 12 for more details on rehabilitation teams and building a working alliance) and to encourage the use of psychological interventions (see Chapters 5–9) with the aim of improving adherence. However, as the research in this area is sparse, researchers are also encouraged to continue to examine the effects of such interventions on rehabilitation adherence.

In Part 2, the five key psychological interventions typically used in sport were outlined and the literature exploring the usefulness of these interventions in sport injury contexts was explored. In addition, a number of practical suggestions on how to use these to facilitate physical and psychosocial recovery were made, an aspect which is undoubtedly one of the unique aspects of this text. All of the chap-ters in Part 2 extended existing literature by the linking of models and theoretical frameworks with the interventions and making them sport injury specific. With respect to goal setting, the most widely adopted of the psychological interventions in rehabilitation, specific types and levels of goals for rehabilitation were suggested. It would be advantageous to explore the usefulness of this framework both in applied and research environments in the future. Similar suggestions were made for imagery where an established model was adapted and applied from sport perform-ance into sport injury rehabilitation settings. Furthermore, this framework could be useful for researchers aiming to explore the use of imagery during rehabilitation in the future, in addition to providing guidance to sport medicine professionals and athletes alike when choosing an appropriate imagery type to meet the desired rehabilitation outcome.

Despite limited empirical evidence from an applied setting, a strong argument was presented to readers for the usefulness of adopting relaxation techniques as an integral part of sport injury rehabilitation. It was recommended that such techniques should be used as a foundation from which other psychological interventions could be built on (for example, imagery). Whilst not a relaxation technique as such, the introduction of mindfulness to sport injury rehabilitation contributed to the contemporary nature of the relaxation chapter. As the application of mindfulness in sport injury rehabilitation is in its infancy, researchers are encouraged to explore mindfulness interventions in the future, particularly its use in managing anxiety, pain and adverse emotions in response to sport injury.

The chapter on self-talk (Chapter 8) introduced the reader to new and innovative concepts. Although existing literature discusses the advantages of positive self-talk over negative self-talk, the current text has explored the importance of considering the interpretation of the content of what is being said, over a simple description of positive/negative and has outlined the key use of 'functional' self-talk during sport injury rehabilitation. That is, when implementing self-talk in rehabilitation, the idea of self-talk being purposeful (motivational or instructional) can be useful in guiding the athlete towards recovery. However, further research in this area is recommended and could focus on the athlete's use of self-talk as part of the rehabilitation process with the aim of seeking further insights into the actual functions of the intervention.

In addition to the four interventions presented above, the value of integrating social support as a key intervention for rehabilitation was presented. Chapter 9 discussed the importance of different types of social support from a range of significant individuals involved with the athlete that can be beneficial during the different phases of rehabilitation. The chapter also described how personal and situational factors that have influence on the athlete impacts on the need for social support. It appears that social support is one of the most researched intervention within sport injury realm, however to understand it fully in the applied settings future research is certainly warranted.

In Part 2 of the book, some key points are worth noting. Firstly, it was emphasised that psychological interventions are most successful if used as part of a wider rehabilitation programme. Secondly, each chapter highlighted a number of key practitioner suggestions, of which a number were directly related to the practical implementation of the interventions. At the core of these suggestions was the need to amalgamate both physical and psychological rehabilitation in such a way that it becomes an accepted part of a holistic sport injury rehabilitation process. Finally, all of the chapters were underpinned by the assumption that all psychological interventions should only be led by professionals who are appropriately skilled and trained to do so.

Following on, Part 3 further emphasised the above. Firstly, Chapter 10 introduced the reader to some of the important practicalities of integrating psychological and physical rehabilitation. Chapter 11 then continued this theme by demonstrating how different members of a rehabilitation team can work together to provide effective holistic recovery. Throughout the book, and particularly in Chapter 11, evidence was provided in support of sport medicine professionals often reporting inadequate training in the psychological aspects of sport injuries. It is the belief of the editors of this text that this is a key area for continued investigation and an area in need of development.

A second novel contribution of this text is the inclusion of the use of counselling skills in sport injury rehabilitation. It was noted that much of the delivery of psychological services in sport (and possibly during rehabilitation) tends to be heavily focused on psychological interventions. It is not disputed that this is a vital component of rehabilitation, as highlighted in Part 2; however, emphasising the importance of the working relationship between the athlete and the practitioner and how such can be facilitated was also deemed important for a number of reasons. Working with an injured athlete might lend itself to the professional knowledge and philosophy of a counselling approach that is underpinned by a process of operating within a trustworthy working alliance and goes far beyond delivering psychological skills alone. Key counselling models have been highlighted and the reader advised of the application of these frameworks when working with injured athletes and how these approaches can then be translated into practice using a set of key counselling skills to build rapport and a working alliance with the injured athlete. Again, it must be pointed out that any practitioner adopting such an approach should have a combination of high levels of self-awareness and the appropriate training.

Finally, Part 3 concluded with a unique chapter on the psychology of physical activity-related injuries, an area currently lacking in empirical research evidence. This chapter applied some of the knowledge from the sport injury research domain and highlighted the need to advance this avenue of investigation further. In society today, there is a clear health promotion agenda encouraging individuals to adopt a more physically active lifestyle. Despite the benefits of adopting such an active lifestyle far outweighing the risks, there is still an increased probability of injury associated with engaging in physical activity. Surprisingly, very little research has been conducted to date focusing on the response to injury in the physically active population. An exciting avenue for future research would include exploring the usefulness of the response to injury frameworks for explaining responses to exercise-related injuries. Furthermore, as we seek to explore enhancing motivation to engage in an active lifestyle, we might consider adopting some theories and practical ideas from this domain and apply them to motivation for rehabilitation. For example, the application of the transtheoretical model to rehabilitation has been proposed as a useful framework; however, this has not yet been empirically explored. The usefulness of active video gaming as a motivational tool for rehabilitation could also be explored in future research.

Despite meeting its aims, this book can be considered a continuation of core texts published 20 years ago and so is still somewhat in its infancy. By providing a description of 'what we know to date', it is hoped that this text will be used to inform practice, to encourage consideration of the implementation of the key suggestions made, as well as serving as a guide for future research by promoting further interest in the area of psychology of sport and physical activity-related injury.

INDEX